# Medical Leadership
# and Management

Geraldine MacCarrick

# Medical Leadership and Management

## A Case-based Approach

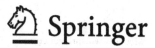 Springer

Geraldine MacCarrick
School of Medicine and Dentistry
James Cook University
Cairns
Queensland
Australia

ISBN 978-1-4471-4747-3     ISBN 978-1-4471-4748-0   (eBook)
DOI 10.1007/978-1-4471-4748-0
Springer London Heidelberg New York Dordrecht

Library of Congress Control Number: 2014949347

Printed on acid-free paper

Springer is part of Springer Science+Business Media (www.springer.com)

# Contents

# Chapter 1
## Introduction

Increasing demands on health care pose ongoing challenges to the health care profession worldwide. Health care managers are called upon to develop new competencies in various domains of their professional practice. Managing and leading health care teams is one of these domains. Management and leadership competence has not traditionally been mandated in undergraduate medical curricula, however increasingly professional medical associations are taking up the challenge of preparing physicians for leadership and management.

Despite lack of formal training, doctors are often invited to take on leadership and management roles in health care. In Australia the Royal Australasian College of Medical Administrators (RACMA) estimates more than 4,000 doctors in public hospital settings are working part time in medical management and clinical leadership roles without necessarily having undergone formal training [1]. Global debate has recently focused on the role of doctors not only to participate in but to lead the required development and transformation of the health services [2], as well as how best to *prepare* future medical leaders [3].

In 1963 the Royal Australasian College of Medical Administrators (RACMA) was established as a college for doctors in senior public sector leadership roles, such as medical superintendents and heads of health services in Australia. The College was recognised by the National Specialist

G. MacCarrick, *Medical Leadership and Management: A Case-based Approach*, DOI 10.1007/978-1-4471-4748-0_1, © Springer-Verlag London 2014

Qualification Advisory Committee in 1980 as the appropriate examining body for the new specialty of medical administration [4]. Since then the College has expanded to include Fellows in Hong Kong and New Zealand [5, 6]. The College now has a well-established training program for doctors specialising in health services management and leadership [4]. The training program has evolved and continues today to be accredited by the Australian Medical Council (AMC) and the Medical Council of New Zealand. In Hong Kong the speciality is known as Administrative Medicine and training is offered through the Hong Kong College of Community Medicine within the Hong Kong Academy of Medicine. The RACMA Medical Leadership and Management Curriculum Framework (Fig. 1.1) provides the basis for the specialist training programs offered by the College.

In the United Kingdom by 1997 the British Association of Medical Managers was well established with 800 members and the Scottish Intercollegiate Initiative in Medical Management was well underway [7]. Lord Darzi's High Quality Care for All: NHS next stage review [8] recommended a mindset change viewing the clinical leader using a "practitioner, partner, leader" model. Similarly other National Health Service in the UK (NHS) and General Medical Council (GMC) publications, for instance Tomorrows Doctors [9], redefine the role of doctor reflecting an international trend to interpret the role more broadly and to include management and leadership as part of this. In 2007, the NHS Institute for Innovation and Improvement was given responsibility for leadership development and building leadership capacity across the NHS. Key amongst the projects that followed was the Enhancing Engagement in Medical Leadership Project to develop and promote medical leadership engagement across the UK. In conjunction with the Academy of Medical Royal Colleges a Medical Leadership Competency Framework (MLCF) was produced [10]. The MLCF provides a structure for the leadership development of medical students, trainees and qualified doctors.

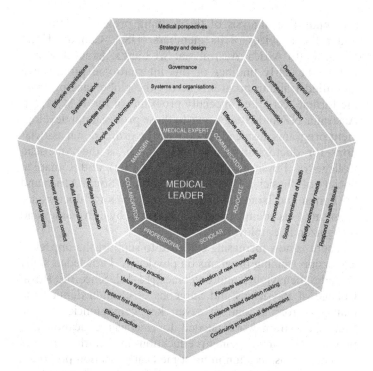

FIGURE 1.1 RACMA medical leadership and management curriculum framework (Reprinted with permission from Royal Australasian College of Medical Administrators)

In Canada the LEADS Framework similarly aims to align and consolidate the leadership competency frameworks and strategies that are found in Canada's health sector [11]. The LEADS Framework, now widely adopted in Canada is a reflection of the key knowledge, skills and attitudes required to lead at all levels of the health care setting. The framework consists of five domains: Lead Self, Engage Others, Achieve Results, Develop Coalitions, and Systems Transformation [12].

In 2012 the World Federation for Medical Managers (WFMM) was established [13] and the same year commenced a comparative analysis of the training programs delivered under the auspices of its members (USA, Canada, Hong Kong, South Africa, Australasia, Sri Lanka, Israel, UK and Italy). The early findings of this international group have identified training programs across the globe ranging from the formal accredited specialty programs of the RACMA in Australia, NZ and Hong Kong, to those professional development programs auspiced for delivery by professional associations for doctors in management (such as the American College of Physician Executives (ACPE)) and Canadian Society of Physician Executives (CSPE). In South Africa and Sri Lanka and Israel management programs for doctors are emerging as academic programs delivered by universities and recognized in employment.

There is now increasing evidence to support the impact of leadership training programs on physicians' knowledge, skills, attitudes, behaviours, and outcomes [14–16]. Since the Royal College of Physicians and Surgeons of Canada defined the managers role as one of seven key competencies in the CanMEDS framework needed for medical education and practice [17], management education in health care has become a consideration in most medical education programs. However, despite these initiatives doctors in training still do not feel fully prepared in terms of perceived leadership competencies [18, 19] suggesting not only room for improved curriculum design to ensure preparedness but also a role for current senior medical managers and leaders as teachers. Medical leaders are well placed to ensure not only a work climate in which education, training and research can flourish but also to take some responsibility for teaching discipline specific competencies related to medical management and leadership.

The following text describes key medical management and leadership competencies using a case based approach. The text and supporting case studies illustrate theoretical and practical aspects of management and leadership in the health care setting.

# References

1. The Royal Australasian College of Medical Administrators. 2014. Available from: http://www.racma.edu.au. Cited 20 Feb 2014.
2. Williams M. Medical managers. Doctors need training in management skills. BMJ. 1997;315(7111):817.
3. Ham C. Strengthening leadership in the NHS. BMJ. 2014;348:1685.
4. The Royal Australasian College of Medical Administrators. Medical Leadership and Management. The Education and Training programs of the Royal Australasian College of Medical Administrators. Curriculum Document. 2011. Available from http://www.rasma.edu.au. Accessed Apr 2014.
5. Jones MR. The first thirty years, 1967–1997, A Chronicle. The Royal Australasian College of Medical Administrators; 1998. Available from http://www.racma.edu.au/index.php?option=com_content&view=article&id=377&Itemid=85.
6. McKimm J, et al. Developing medical leadership: a comparative review of approaches in the UK and New Zealand. Int J Leadersh Public Serv. 2009;5(3):10–24.
7. Simpson J, Smith R. Why healthcare systems need medical managers. BMJ. 1997;314(7095):1636.
8. Darzi A. King Edward's Hospital Fund for London. High quality care for all: NHS next stage review final report – summary, London, King's Fund. 2008.
9. General Medical Council, G. Tomorrow's doctors – outcomes and standards for undergraduate medical education. 2009. Available from: http://www.gmc-uk.org/education/undergraduate/tomorrows_doctors.asp. Accessed 20 Feb 2014.
10. The Academy of Medical Royal Colleges and the NHS Institute for Innovation and Improvement. Medical leadership competency framework. 2011. Available from: http://www.leadershipacademy.nhs.uk/wp-content/uploads/2012/11/NHSLeadership-Leadership-Framework-Medical-Leadership-Competency-Framework-3rd-ed.pdf.
11. Snell AJ, Briscoe D, Dickson G. From the inside out: the engagement of physicians as leaders in health care settings. Qual Health Res. 2011;21(7):952–67.
12. The LEADS Collaborative. 2013. Available from: http://www.leadersforlife.ca/. Accessed Apr 2014.

13. World Federation for Medical Managers. Available from: http://www.wfmm.org/. Accessed Mar 2014.
14. Straus S, Soobiah C, Levinson W. The impact of leadership training programs on physicians in Academic Medical Centers: a systematic review. Acad Med. 2013;88(5):710–23.
15. Day DV. Leadership development: a review in context. Leadersh Q. 2000;11(4):581.
16. Hemmer PR, et al. Leadership and management training for residents and fellows: a curriculum for future medical directors. Arch Pathol Lab Med. 2007;131(4):610–4.
17. Frank J, Danoff D. The CanMEDS initiative: implementing an outcomes-based framework of physician competencies. Med Teach. 2007;29(7):642–7.
18. Berkenbosch L, et al. Medical residents' perceptions of their competencies and training needs in health care management: an international comparison. BMC Med Educ. 2013;13:25.
19. Schoenmaker SG, et al. Victorian junior doctors' perception of their competency and training needs in healthcare management. Aust Health Rev. 2013;37(4):412–7.

# Chapter 2
## Professional Leadership and Management in Medicine

**Abstract**  As health care leaders, doctors need to be strategic leaders demonstrating the ability to anticipate, envision and to empower others to create change. Within this context health care leaders need to demonstrate awareness of ethical and professional issues in managerial decision making.

**Keywords**  Ethics • Ethical decision making • Professionalism • Emotional intelligence • Continuing professional development

## Professional Leader

Across the globe medical managers are being asked to undertake a challenging yet pivotal role, in demonstrating effective leadership to bring about real improvements in clinical care and health management in health care services. As health care leaders, doctors need to be strategic leaders demonstrating the ability to anticipate, envision and to empower others to create change [1]. Strategic leaders need to be able to determine the strategic direction of the organisation, develop its human capital and sustain an effective organisational culture. Within this context health care leaders need to demonstrate awareness of ethical and professional issues in managerial decision making. Ethical leadership creates a

G. MacCarrick, *Medical Leadership and Management:*
*A Case-based Approach*, DOI 10.1007/978-1-4471-4748-0_2,
© Springer-Verlag London 2014

work environment in which ethical behaviours are rewarded and in which all people are treated with dignity.

The relevant competencies, i.e. knowledge skills attitudes and behaviours required of professional leader include:

- Implementing management decisions which are ethically appropriate
- Consistently acting with integrity and accountability
- Demonstrating respect for professional, legal and ethical codes of practice
- Demonstrating maintenance of professional competence and lifelong learning such as participating in peer review and audits
- Demonstrating willingness to accept constructive feedback
- Demonstrating a balance between personal and professional priorities
- Recognising other professionals in need and responding appropriately
- Demonstrating emotionally intelligent leadership and reflective practice
- Demonstrates knowledge of current leadership theory and reflects this in practice

One of the key distinctions identified in the literature is the distinction between leadership and management. Leadership is about setting direction and influencing and motivating others to achieve change. Management on the other hand, is concerned with assembling and organising resources to achieve organisational goals. The current literature sees leading and managing as separate but complementary activities.

To effectively lead in health care, the modern health care leader should have knowledge of current leadership frameworks and theories as they pertain to everyday practice. The National Health Service (NHS) (UK) Leadership Qualities Framework is an evidenced based leadership framework created following substantial research targeting the specific needs of the health care environment. In Canada the LEADS Framework similarly aims to align and consolidate the leadership competency frameworks and strategies that are found in Canada's health sector.

Leadership theories have developed through four distinct phases. In the first half of the twentieth century the *trait theories* prevailed. These theories tried to identify intellectual emotional physical and other personal traits which appeared to differentiate between successful and unsuccessful leaders. Trait theories however showed no consistent pattern of predicting effective leadership performance and it is now recognised that leadership is a far more complex phenomenon and not just based on traits. (Nonetheless it is worth noting that trait theory has had a recent resurgence of interest with Goleman's work on emotional intelligence [2]). From the 1950s onwards the focus of leadership theories moved away from personal traits to *behavioural theories*. Blake and Mouton explored concern for task and concern for people along the X and Y axes of what they called a "managerial grid" [3]. The underlying premise of this and other models is that leadership behaviours can be consciously selected and modified at will. Behavioural theories of leadership nonetheless failed to identify the sorts of behaviours that worked in particular situations. This aspect was further developed by the *contingency or situation theories* of leadership. Hersey and Blanchard's situational leadership model [4], for example asserts that the leader needs to adapt their leadership style depending on the competence and commitment of their followers. Fiedler's contingency model [5] specifies that performance is contingent upon both the leaders motivational system and the degree to which the leader controls and influences the situation. Contingency variables in this model include leader member relations (that is trust confidence and respect that followers have for the leader); task structure (that is the extent to which a task performed by employees is routine or non-routine) and position power (that is the extent to which the leader has reward, coercive and legitimate power for hiring firing and promotion). Fiedler's contingency model uses the least preferred co- worker (LPC) scale as a measure of leadership style. It indicates whether a leader describes their least preferred co-worker in negative or positive terms. Low – LPC leaders tend to be task oriented, that is the focus on improving relationships with subordinates is only *after* they are assured that tasks have been completed. High – LPC leaders first concentrate on establishing good relationships with their subordinates and then focus on task completion. Since the 1980s the focus of leadership theories has shifted to consider how leaders can best manage the context of continuous change.

Change is an ongoing process within most healthcare settings. The health care leader needs to be familiar with theories of organisational change [6, 7] as well as practical approaches to dealing with resistance to change [8]. Transformational leaders release human potential by empowering others. New leadership constructs such as 'authentic leadership' [9, 10] claim a global ethical meltdown in leadership calling for leadership that is both 'authentic' and 'positive'. Researchers and academics cite several components to authentic leadership including self- awareness, self- development and a positive moral perspective.

## Self Awareness and Reflective Practice

Self-awareness is at the core of personal and professional development. Being able to recognise one's skills, strengths and weaknesses, as well as the impact one has on those around helps develop leadership potential. Self-awareness includes a recognition of individual strengths and weaknesses, as well as a high level of self-concept and a stable sense of self knowledge and self belief [11]. The literature on authentic leadership suggest the importance of transparency in expressing emotions and feelings to others, whilst at the same time regulating such emotions to minimise displays of inappropriate or potentially harmful emotions [12]. Emotional Intelligence is the ability to understand what you are feeling and why, and to perceive emotions in others. Leaders with an internal focus of control are aware of how they impact on others, both positively and negatively [13]. The ability to recognise and regulate this information in productive ways is important in the delivery of health care in highly complex organisational structures.

Soliciting feedback from those we trust is an important means of increasing self-awareness. Although feedback is normally understood to mean a formal process that happens infrequently, it can be more effective if delivered more informally and frequently. Self-reflection also helps ensure actions taken are evidence based. There are many ways to reflect, some of these include – journal writing; 'thinking out loud'; recording reflections on a tape or meditation. Maintaining a journal is a particularly useful way to become more aware of one's own practice, recognize patterns of events and individual response to these. Journaling can also help identify learning needs and enable linkages to be made between theory and practice. One outcome of the reflective journal may be a Personal Development Plan (PDP). The latter is designed to enable the health care manager with the help and support of a mentor to assess his/her own effectiveness in the current role, identify future goals and set objectives to improve current performance. Developing a PDP consists of conducting a personal evaluation, meeting with a mentor to discuss a plan and continuous review. The sorts of considerations such a plan may contain might include a reflection on the skills, knowledge and personal qualities required for the current role (which do you possess/in which areas would you like to improve/what additional skills do you feel you need to help realise your future aspirations?). In articulating goals it is important to make them specific, measurable, appropriate, realistic and time-bound.

Reflecting on one's own performance (rather than someone else's) requires personal insight; the skills of self-assessment and the ability to accept and act upon feedback from peers. Reflective observation is described as the second stage of the Lewin/Kolb learning cycle [14]. Kolb suggests that there are four stages which follow from each other. Concrete experience is followed by reflection on that experience on a personal basis. This may then be followed by the derivation of general rules describing that experience, or the application of theory to practice (Abstract Conceptualisation), and then to developing ways of modifying the next occasion of that experience (Active Experimentation). Schön (1983) suggested that the capacity to reflect on action in order to seek continuous improvement is one of the defining characteristics of professional practice [15]. Evidence of reflective practice as health care leaders includes participation in self – directed learning such as peer review and audit. Professional leadership also requires the demonstrated ability to accept constructive feedback and the preparedness to change behaviour as appropriate, based on such feedback. Porter-O'Grady and Malloch [16] suggest leaders increase their self-awareness by asking themselves the following simple questions on a daily basis: What difference did I make today? Who did I affect? What opportunities did I miss? What do I need to change?

In their original discussions on authentic leadership, Luthans and Avolio [10] identified that authentic leaders display confidence, optimism, hope and resilience. These capacities often spring from a balance between our professional and personal lives. The key to managing oneself, one's job and one's life is about understanding oneself and setting priorities. A quote from British (Canadian-born) physician and mentor Sir William Osler over a hundred years ago captures the importance of achieving that essential balance:

> *While medicine is to be your vocation, or calling, see to it that you have also an avocation – some intellectual pastime which may serve to keep you in touch with the world of art, of science, or of letters. Sir William Osler, from After Twenty-Five Years, in Aequanimitas.*

Underpinning most leadership constructs is a requirement for a strong moral and ethical framework. Medical practitioners are expected to act at all times within the ethical and professional code set out for the profession. As medical managers there is a need for heightened awareness of the ethical issues in managerial as well as clinical decision making. Specific areas of competency include an understanding of medical ethics, awareness of conflict of interest, recognising one's own strengths and weaknesses, understanding the legal and ethical responsibilities of a medical practitioner and consistently acting with integrity. The professional medical manager is also required to be capable of identifying breaches of professionalism in other colleagues and responding to these appropriately. Where there is concern in relation to potentially unsafe systems, the medical leader must act to prevent any immediate risk to patient safety by taking appropriate action.

## Making Sense of Our World

A key aspect that influences interaction with others and may affect communication with colleagues and patients is how we make sense of our world. Heider [17] claims there is a strong need to understand events in the world around us by attributing them to people and/or the environment. He argued that we make continual causal analyses about other's behaviours where the behaviour is either attributed to the person's disposition or external situational factors. Attributions are only inferences and therefore prone to bias. Chris Argyris developed the ladder of inference in 1990 as a tool to understand the thinking process and help us understand how and why we think as we do about an issue [18].

There are several questionnaires and self-discovery tools to help the medical manager inform this process including the Myers Briggs Personality Questionnaire [19]; Belbin's Team Type Questionnaire [20] and Learning Styles Questionnaire [21]. Perhaps the most widely used test for typing personality in organisational settings today is the Myers-Briggs Type Indicator (MBTI) [22]. This instrument is based on the concept of psychological type developed by Jung in the 1920s. From Jung's work Myers and Briggs identified four basic aspects of personality: where we get our energy, what we attend to, how we make decisions and how we operate in the world. Most sit at any point between the two extremes on these dichotomies. The Extraversion–Introversion dichotomy; the Sensing–Intuition dichotomy; the Thinking–Feeling dichotomy and the Judgment–Perception dichotomy. Using this inventory individuals can be classified on either end of the four dichotomies, giving 16 possible psychological types which indicate where preferences lie. The types are designated by the appropriate letter from each dimension: e.g. an ESTJ is an Extroverted, Sensate, Thinking Judger, while an INFP is an Introverted, Intuitive, Feeling Perceiver. Whilst the MBTI has become a very popular staff development tool, caution is needed in interpretation. Although we do tend to have a natural preference for one or the other end of the dichotomies, we can all demonstrate some of the eight preferences at different times. The Myers-Briggs indicator is therefore best viewed as a useful adjunct to help team members in the workplace understand how we may view the world a little differently from others, thereby facilitating team work and avoiding potential conflict.

In summary leadership in health care requires strategic vision, professionalism, high levels of self-awareness and commitment to ethical practice. Leadership also requires commitment to fostering a culture in which all people are treated with dignity and respect.

## Case Study 1

You are new to this regional hospital and have recently accepted a new post as Director of Clinical Training. As part of this portfolio you are responsible for all junior doctor education and training matters as well as maintaining your clinical portfolio (as an Emergency Physician 3 days a week).

You are heartened by the welcome you have received from the CEO and Director of Medical Services (DMS). As you take up residence in your new office you see posters along the corridor as you approach the Clinical Training Unit supporting family friendly policies and the safe working hours campaign for junior doctors. After the first month has passed you begin to notice an increasing trend of being "copied in" on emails from the CEO and the DMS pertaining to a wide range of hospital management issues not just junior doctor matters. This is also occurring after hours, on weekends and when the CEO is travelling. Many of the emails sent from her Blackberry© are being responded to by other colleagues before the next working day and you feel obliged to do the same. You also observe a habit of setting early morning or late afternoon meetings. You are committed to supporting a safe culture amongst junior doctors and this was particularly emphasised at your selection interview but you feel this is now at odds with the behaviour you yourself are beginning to demonstrate.

## As a New Member of the Executive Team, How Will You Manage This Situation?

Consider the following.

- What is the local culture at this hospital?, i.e. the sets of values, beliefs and behaviours that govern particular behaviours. Why is this so?
- Authentic leadership relates to the alignment between internal values and external behaviour. What are your values?
- How might this work practice impact on your vision for safe practice amongst junior doctors? What message does it send?
- Are the CEO's values consistent with her own actions? How might you explore this? Is there a possibility she may be unaware of the mismatch?
- Discuss with other colleagues. Is this a practice of responding to emails and meeting scheduling which is new or has it become entrenched? Do others share your concerns?
- Consider how to prepare the case for change.

- Remain politically astute. What is happening inside the organisation/team? What can and cannot be achieved, setting appropriate priorities and timelines.
- What things can you do each day to encourage your own reflectivity?

# References

1. Hitt MA, Ireland RD, Hoskisson RE. Strategic management: competitiveness and globalization: concepts. 8th ed. Mason: South-Western; 2009. xxv, 389, I–26 p.
2. Goleman D. Emotional intelligence, why it can matter more than IQ. London: Bloomsbury; 2004.
3. Blake R, Mouton J. The managerial grid III: a new look at the classic that has boosted productivity and profits for thousands of corporations worldwide. Houston: Gulf Pub. Co. Book Division; 1985.
4. Hersey P, Blanchard KH. Management of organizational behavior: utilizing human resources. 3rd ed. Englewood Cliffs: Prentice-Hall; 1977.
5. Fiedler FE, Garcia JE. New approaches to effective leadership – cognitive resources and organisational performance. New York: Wiley; 1987.
6. Lewin K, Cartwright D. Field theory in social science: selected theoretical papers. London: Tavistock; 1952.
7. Gersick CJG. Revolutionary change theories: a multi-level exploration of the punctuated equilibrium paradigm. Acad Manage Rev. 1991;16(1):10–36.
8. Kotter JP, Schlesinger LA. Choosing strategies for change. Harv Bus Rev. 2008;86(7/8):130–9.
9. Avolio BJ, Gardner WL, Walumbwa FO, May D. Unlocking the mask: a look at the process by which authentic leaders impact follower attitudes and behaviours. Leadersh Q. 2004;15(6):801–23.
10. Luthans F, Avolio BJ. Authentic leadership: a positive development approach. In: Cameron K, Dutton JE, Quinn RE, editors. Positive organisational scholarship. San Francisco: Berrett-Koehler; 2003.
11. Shamir B, Eilam G. "What's your story?" A life-stories approach to authentic leadership development. Leadersh Q. 2005;16(3):395–417.

12. Gardner WL, et al. "Can you see the real me?" A self-based model of authentic leader and follower development. Leadersh Q. 2005;16(3):343–72.

13. Hughes M, Terrell JB. Emotional intelligence in action. 2nd ed. Hoboken: Wiley; 2011.

14. Kolb DA. Experiential learning: experience as the source of learning and development. Englewood Cliffs: Prentice-Hall; 1984. xiii, 256 p.

15. Schön DA. The reflective practitioner: how professionals think in action. New York: Basic Books; 1983. x, 374 p.

16. Porter-O'Grady T, Malloch K. Quantum leadership: a textbook of new leadership. Sudbury: Jones and Bartlett; 2003. xiii, 377 p.

17. Heider F, Benesh-Weiner M. Fritz Heider: the notebooks. New York: München-Weinheim; 1987.

18. Argyris C. The applicability of organizational sociology. London: Cambridge University Press; 1972. ix, 138 p.

19. Myers I, Kirby L, Myers K. Introduction to type: a guide to understanding your results on the Myers-Briggs Type Indicator. 6th ed. Palo Alto: Consulting Psychologists Press; 1998. iii, 43.

20. Belbin RM. Team roles at work. Oxford/Boston: Butterworth-Heinemann; 1993. vii, 152.

21. Samarakoon LF, Fernando T, Rodrigo C. Learning styles and approaches to learning among medical undergraduates and postgraduates. BMC Med Educ. 2013;13:42.

22. Myers IB, Mccaulley MH, Most R. Manual, a guide to the development and use of the Myers-Briggs type indicator. Palo Alto, Ca: Consulting Psychologists Press; 1985.

# Chapter 3
## The Effective Medical Manager

**Abstract** The effective medical manager is expected to plan and manage organisations and the people within them utilising available resources appropriately. The medical manager brings clinical input to organisational decision making.

**Keywords** Organisational behaviour • Prioritising tasks • Manage time effectively • 'Systems approach' to management • Health financing models • Human resource management

## Effective Management

The effective health care leader is expected to plan and manage organisations and the people within them utilising available resources appropriately. The role of the medical manager is to bring medical input to organisational decision making. It is expected that the doctor has expert knowledge of the health care system organisation and funding and can manage in order to produce the best results for patients, doctors and other staff. It is also expected she/he will understand the relevant jurisdictional health care systems and be familiar with national health and funding priorities.

G. MacCarrick, *Medical Leadership and Management:*
*A Case-based Approach*, DOI 10.1007/978-1-4471-4748-0_3,
© Springer-Verlag London 2014

The key relevant competencies, required of an effective medical manager include:

- Demonstrates a knowledge of organisational behaviour
- Demonstrates effective management within a business environment
- Demonstrates the ability to prioritise tasks and manage time effectively
- Identifies and understands all interrelated processes in a 'systems approach' to management
- Understands health financing models
- Develops and implements budgets for decision making
- Implements appropriate human resource management strategies including recruitment, allocation and monitoring of human resources
- Understands the principles of preparing and critiquing business cases, audits, financial statements and cost benefit analyses
- Understands the principles of allocating finite resources appropriately

The health care system organisation is a complex one. In the last decade the increasing demands on health care delivery across the globe have had significant impact on the structure of health care systems and strategies for care reform. Increased consumer expectations and the demand for cost effective and efficient health care by health care funders coupled with government demand for increased accountability and transparency have contributed to this [1]. Over the last two decades, a range of policy initiatives have also been introduced to improve accountability of health care organisations and these have included a more managed approach to health care and a range of initiatives to address concerns over patient safety and reducing clinical error.

## Service Planning

Hospitals usually operate within a network delivering a range of health services provided by either the hospital and/or a variety of health care centres or units. Hospital services are typically grouped around the following: inpatient; outpatient; emergency; community; mental health; aged care; public health and health promotion. These health care facilities vary in terms of service capabilities and include community health centres, regional hospitals, tertiary hospitals and specialised health services. Typically each jurisdiction has a health services plan which provides overarching direction and guidance detailing proposed reforms, strategies for funding and the necessary infrastructure, workforce and assets to deliver these reforms. Health services plans ensure that the services deliver according to demand and make effective use of available resources. The medical manager is expected to participate in health services planning, providing overarching direction to departmental plans. As such the medical manager will need to be cognisant of the service capability of his/her organisation and be familiar with strategies for funding, workforce planning and infrastructure. Service delivery also needs to be aligned with legislation, regulations, standards, policies and frameworks, and relevant medical college training standards.

In addition to service planning medical managers are typically involved directly with capital infrastructure planning and development, for example providing support to districts and departments undertaking local or specific planning projects. Such support can include careful consideration and advocacy for dedicated space for clinical training requirements (such as Clinical Skills laboratories or affiliated university teaching space) as well as clinical service delivery.

## Human Resource Management

Human Resource Management (HRM) functions are an integral part of the medical manager's role. Guest describes HRM as comprising a set of policies "designed to maximise organisational integration, employee commitment, flexibility and quality of work" [2]. Progressive HRM relies on active staff participation and heavy investment in training and career development as well as flexible work patterns. HRM to be effective needs to be strategic and linked to the overall strategy of the organisation.

A thorough understanding of theoretical underpinnings of productivity and work motivation [3–7] will help the medical manager guide job design and planning. Essentially staff satisfaction is a multidimensional construct [8] and needs to be fully understood by the medical manager. If employee performance and valued rewards are linked in some way, work motivation and improved productivity can be expected to follow. Ideally work should be designed such that staff are utilising their knowledge and skills; have the necessary information to be able to fulfil their jobs; have had appropriate training and development; have the opportunity to enhance existing skills; are able to anticipate problems and participate in the solution and are encouraged to participate in decision making processes. All of these aspects will determine how employees perceive and perform their work and interact with other work colleagues. These factors will also impact upon recruitment, appraisal, reward (i.e. remuneration) and development.

Although in most health care settings many aspects of recruitment and selection are delegated nonetheless the medical manager needs to be familiar with the relevant processes for the associated tasks such as identifying need for a vacant position, advertising, seeking approval to fill positions, forming interview panels, shortlisting, selection processes, criminal history checking, completion of selection reports, referee reports and relevant health checks (including vaccination requirements). The manager should also be familiar with the processes for appointing emergent short term placements, for example using locum agencies.

A particular consideration for the medical manager is the global nature of the medical workforce. When appointing international medical graduates a series of additional checks are generally required. Typically the medical manager becomes involved in decisions such as whether the position is deemed necessary in the first place and whether the particular post is recruitable locally prior to advertising overseas. Sufficient time must be allowed for the completion of the necessary processes for overseas appointments. This can take several months and includes checking certified copies of Curriculum Vitaes, medical degrees and proof of identity. Confirmation of language proficiency is also an additional concern for the medical manager.

An important aspect of HRM for the medical manager is credentialing and defining scope of clinical practice. In most jurisdictions registered medical practitioners require periodic peer review of their credentials and scope of clinical practice by a relevant committee. Credentials represent the formal qualifications, training, experience and clinical competence of the medical practitioner and scope of clinical practice (also referred to as 'clinical privileges') that a practitioner may exercise at a specific facility. Health care facilities have a legal responsibility to ensure the safety and quality of the health care provided by employed medical practitioners and it is typically the role of the senior medical manager to oversee this. The rapid expansion of clinical services, potential procedures and medical equipment makes it even more important to safeguard patients from any associated risk.

Credentialing policies and practices are subject to natural justice and should be fair and transparent. Credentialing should be informed by the respective service's health services strategic plan (as above) and therefore be reviewed regularly as service demands change over time. The medical manager's role specifically is to ensure that a credentialing and scope of clinical practice process is in place in her/his jurisdiction and maintain and retain appropriate records.

In terms of remuneration, salary levels are typically defined within the instrument of an award, however medical managers should be familiar with the relevant entitlements for their staff. This includes pay scales and allowances. In addition the manager needs to be fluent in relevant employment conditions such implementation of flexible and improved working initiatives such as family friendly provisions; job sharing arrangements and medical fatigue risk management. Regular consultation with staff as well as exit surveys conducted on termination of employment, are a useful way to identify views about conditions of employment including training opportunities, remuneration and benefits. Such feedback can assist in design and implementation of improvement strategies.

Performance Management helps ensure employees have clear objectives and work expectations with plans for self-development. An integral part of every medical manager's responsibility therefore is to meet regularly with staff and identify performance objectives as well the support required to achieve these objectives. Performance appraisal and development is usually mandated for all employees except those on short term and temporary contracts. A typical performance appraisal and development cycle consists of drafting an initial agreement which sets out performance targets and professional development needs; supporting performance and developmental activities over time, making adjustments to performance targets if appropriate, followed by performance and appraisal and review. The latter consists of an examination of progress against developmental activities and setting out performance goals for the next review cycle.

In recent times there has been significant development in the field of monitoring the performance of doctors by regulatory bodies such as Medical Councils which have the responsibility of monitoring the performance of doctors within their jurisdiction. In the United Kingdom, the General Medical Council (GMC) has introduced a process of regular revalidation for doctors by a responsible officer. Typically the responsible officer will be a senior medical manager in the organisation in which the doctor works. As part of this process active clinicians must secure a continuing licence to practise on the grounds that they have demonstrated they are "up to date and fit to practise" medicine [9]. Senior medical managers are expected to be involved in this process of revalidation and have oversight of it. Multisource feedback has been increasingly used to provide valuable information about doctors' performance. The process consists of obtaining feedback from subordinates, peers, and supervisors as a means by which managers might encourage improved performance. Multisource feedback has become a central component of most models of revalidation. Care must be taken when interpreting multisource feedback. Recent studies highlight the need for guidance for doctors when collating appropriate samples of feedback from colleagues and patients, and, importantly, the need for guidance for those responsible for interpreting and responding to feedback on doctors' professionalism [10–12].

As part of this process the medical manager should be familiar with the processes in place to address ongoing poor performance, serious issues and misconduct. The principles guiding identified poor work performance include early intervention, provision of appropriate training and associated resources to support the employee, monitoring of performance and provision of constructive feedback and counselling. The key is constructive feedback. There is now convincing evidence that systematic feedback delivered by a credible source can change and improve clinical performance [13].

If these measures fail then action should be taken which is based on procedural fairness, objectivity and accountability. In some situations it may be necessary to formally investigate and at times disciplinary action is required. Such circumstances would include criminal activity or use of substances adversely affecting the practitioners' clinical competence; misconduct or absence without approval of leave.

Medical managers have a responsibility to know their legal obligations to employees. An important consideration when rostering doctors for example, is the legal obligation to provide a safe system of work including safe work scheduling. The relevant Occupational Health and Safety Acts will describe employers' responsibilities in this regard. Increased awareness of the effects of fatigue for instance has necessitated several initiatives to ensure patient safety by creating a more sustainable workforce. Doctors are particularly prone to fatigue. Hospital and community based practice often necessitates shift work and extended hours to maintain service provision, however it is now well recognised that disruption of circadian rhythm can exacerbate the effects of fatigue. Studies have shown that performance impairment at 18 h of sustained wakefulness is equivalent to a blood alcohol concentration >0.05 % [14, 15]

Apart from the implications for safety and quality, fatigue can also contribute to poor morale, absenteeism and sick leave. Addressing medical workforce fatigue has become an important priority for many hospitals and the medical manager plays a key role in this.

The manager has a responsibility to institute and uphold relevant policies with respect to fatigue awareness and to be familiar with resources available to assist with risk assessment. Several research groups have developed models for estimating the work-related fatigue associated with shift work. One of these models, the Fatigue Audit InterDyne (FAID), can be used to quantify the work-related fatigue associated with any duty schedule using hours of work as the sole input [15].

## Managers and Funding

Medical managers require an understanding of the health funding models such as Activity Based Funding which operate in many jurisdictions. These are designed to ensure that distribution of health care resources is more efficient, effective and equitable in relation to population health needs and activity. Case-mix (CM) measurement for example categorizes patients according to perceived need for service or resource use. The aim of CM measurement is to develop an equitable distribution of resources across a particular client group. One of the earliest approaches for grouping patient was developed in the acute care sector and uses primary diagnosis as the main method of classification. These groups, known as Diagnosis-Related Groups (DRGs), categorize patients into unique groups that share similar processes of care and would be expected to receive a similar set of services or interventions [16]. With the introduction of newer funding models it is important to capture all activity.

Medical managers who have oversight of clinical data collection must ensure it is clear, comprehensive and concise. Funding models may contain funding incentives and disincentives (penalties) such as incentives for timely submission of clinical coding and data reporting and penalties for late submission of coded data. To be effective the medical manager needs to be familiar with these internal processes and advise staff accordingly. Managers also need to be familiar with their local budget process. The aim of the budget process is to provide budget certainty for budget holders through the full allocation of known resources in advance. If additional funding is required the usual process is to submit a business case. Business cases should be specific about what the requested funding is to be used for. Linking the case with existing service related plans, it is important to detail how the funding proposal will deliver on current priorities. The proposal should also identify any links to identified health reform agreements and associated targets. Costing assumptions should make clear how the costs were derived (e.g. numbers of new staff or building or refurbishment required). A well-developed business case will typically include performance targets to measure the effectiveness of the initiative and will identify outputs under the relevant business funding model. It is important to consider the timing of funding submissions. For example the requested funds will need to be cash flowed across the appropriate number of years if it is a multi-year proposal.

## Time Management

Effective time management is an essential tool of the successful medical manager. Common time wasting activities include unscheduled meetings, interruptions, telephone calls, lack of planning, crisis management and insufficient information to complete a task. As a medical manager it is key to allocate sufficient time to plan. Reflecting on objectives and goals will ensure they remain *SMART* [17], *i.e., S*pecific; *M*easurable; *Attainable; R*ealistic and *T*ime-bound. When George Doran first documented the SMART acronym in 1981, he intended the term *specific* to refer to targeting a specific area for improvement; *measurable* to suggest an indicator of progress, *assignable* to specify who will do it; *realistic* to refer to what results can realistically be achieved given available resources and *time-related* to refer to identifying when the results can be achieved.

Scheduling regular 'blocked time' without interruptions in the daily calendar of a manager will ensure more is accomplished. Avoiding tight scheduling will increase efficiency. A well briefed executive support officer to manage the daily calendar will ensure allocation of time for outside meeting activities such as accumulating paperwork and mail. A dedicated support officer can also assist with research and preparation of rough drafts of reports if correct delegation is used.

In summary, the medical manager makes regular decisions about allocating finite resources. The ability to prioritize tasks and effectively manage time and to actively engage colleagues, patients and carers as integral participants in the decision-making process is critical. Oversight of an effective human resource management strategy will ensure integration, commitment, flexibility and quality of work.

## Case Study 1

You have recently commenced as Director of Medical Services of a rural hospital and this is your first rural posting. Towards the end of the Welcome Reception held at the nearby township's main hotel, the hospital's only specialist Urologist, has asked to meet with you urgently the following day to discuss renewal of her contract. You try to remain friendly and in the spirit of the evening however she remains insistent and monopolizes your attention. The CEO finally succeeds in 'extricating' you from the situation and promises to apprise you of the situation in the near future, "when you have had time to settle in". You decide to tidy a few last minute things in the office on the way home and whilst there pull out the Urologist's contract in advance of the next morning's meeting. You discover that the same Urologist has had several email discussions with your predecessor regarding renewal of her contract which is due to expire in under a year. It appears no conclusion had been reached. You also find no evidence of any performance management or evidence of any credentialing committee having been convened to oversee an escalating number of new procedures being carried out by this urologist. At the meeting the following day you advise the Urologist of the need for more time to consider her request. She expresses her displeasure saying she understood from your predecessor that her re-appointment was a 'matter of course'. Pushed by her abrasive attitude you finally allude to the possible need to review scope of practice given the large number of new procedures being carried out. She becomes irate threatening to withdraw her service to the hospital in advance of her contract term and insisting she wants to take this matter further to the CEO and the Board.

**What are the issues here?**
**How will you manage the situation in the short term?**
**In the long term?**
Consider the following:

- This is your first 'assignment'
- Take time to collect the facts, what can you ascertain about what has been agreed to in the past, how much still relevant? Was there potential for misunderstanding? Obtain the CEOs input.
- Was performance review done in the past?
- What information available for e.g. patient complaints, compliments, audits, morbidity and mortality outcomes, past credentialing processes etc.?
- How to align appointments process with hospital's service plan
- Manage threat to withdraw services – raises potential for breach of contract

- What legislation concerning employment and industrial law do you need to consult?
- What arrangements are currently in place at this hospital for credentialing and are these policies being adhered to?
- If poor compliance with the credentialing policy is it due to technical issues such as inadequate IT systems such as easily searchable databases, lack of consistent templates and processes or is it a change management issue
- Document the entire process carefully

## Case Study 2

You are the Director of Medical Services of a large teaching hospital that provides general and specialty medical and surgical services. It is the regional hub for cardiothoracic surgery, neurosurgery, neonatal intensive care and high risk obstetrics. You have just met with the Dean of the affiliated medical school as part of your regular partnership agreement stakeholder meetings. Towards the end of the discussion, when the others have left the meeting room the Dean mentions a "rather sensitive matter". Medical students on the surgery rotation have consistently expressed concerns in the end of term evaluations that the Deputy Head of Surgery is often vague and confused during the tutorials and seems to be 'getting worse'. He recently tripped whilst delivering a lecture, narrowly missing the lectern then left the lecture hall without explanation and did not return.

You immediately check the surgeon's file and see he is due to retire in a year, after 30 years of loyal service to the hospital and the medical school. You discuss the case with the Head of Surgery who assures you that the doctor is just "getting on" but is still a good clinician and he is happy to let him continue his regular list as long as the senior registrar is available to assist, when one is available. He acknowledges he has heard the students' complaints but cannot assign anyone else to the teaching role as he is chronically short-staffed. The

Head of Surgery has made no effort to investigate or act on previous complaints.

**What are the key issues?**
**How will you manage this situation?**
Consider the following:

- Meet again with Dean to establish the facts
- Ascertain details of relationship with the Medical School, and shared responsibility for performance management of staff member
- Potentially impaired medical practitioner
- Patient safety
- Performance management system
- Performance management of Departmental Head
- Seek HR advice
- Procedural fairness and natural justice
- Role of HOD, care not to usurp the HOD's role however if no action forthcoming consider setting up meeting with Deputy Head of Surgery with HOD to discuss
- Audit of patient charts
- Review policy for performance management of medical staff
- Implement training for clinical directors and senior staff in performance management
- Review of clinical director's effectiveness, performance and training
- Investigate options for wellness program for medical practitioners

# Case Study 3

You are the director of Clinical Training at a regional hospital. A junior resident approaches you for support and to discuss his upcoming appearance before the coroner's Court. As the junior resident discusses the case in which he was directly involved, it becomes obvious that he has been working unusually long shifts. The resident also advises that he has heard the Medical Association have been invited to give evidence at the proceedings. You feel certain that the issue of safe working hours at your hospital will be considered as part of the hearing.

**What are the key issues?**
**How will you manage these in the short term?**
**In the long term?**
Consider the following:

- manage confidentiality issues
- support for junior resident, a first appearance at the Coroner's Court can cause significant distress
- involve senior executive in review of safe working hours at your hospital
- education and training around workplace occupational health and safety
- identify champions of safe working hours campaign
- raise awareness of adverse consequences to patients and staff as a result of fatigue
- Consider models for estimating the work-related fatigue associated with shift work at this hospital
- Anticipate Medical Association response to hearing
- Prepare to manage media

# References

1. Porter ME, Teisberg EO. Redefining health care: creating value-based competition on results. Boston: Harvard Business School Press; 2006.
2. Guest DE. Human resource management and industrial relations. J Manag Stud. 1987;24(5):503–21.
3. Maslow AH. A theory of human motivation. Psychol Rev. 1943;50(4):370–96.
4. Herzberg F, Mausner B, Snyderman BB. The motivation to work. New York: Wiley; 1959.
5. McClelland DC. The achieving society. New York: Van Nostrand; 1961.
6. McGregor D. The human side of enterprise. New York: McGraw-Hill; 1960. p. 246.

7. Vroom VH, Deci EL. Management and motivation: selected readings. In: Penguin modern management readings. Harmondsworth: Penguin; 1970. p. 399.

8. Krueger P, Brazil K, Lohfeld L, Edward HG, Lewis D, Tjam E. Organization specific predictors of job satisfaction: findings from a Canadian multi-site quality of work life cross-sectional survey. BMC Health Serv Res. 2002;2(1):6.

9. Rubin P. Commentary: the role of appraisal and multisource feedback in the UK General Medical Council's new revalidation system. Acad Med. 2012;87(12):1654–6.

10. Hall W, et al. Assessment of physician performance in Alberta: the physician achievement review. CMAJ. 1999;161(1):52–7.

11. Campbell JL, Roberts M, Wright C, Hill J, Greco M, Taylor M, Richards S. Factors associated with variability in the assessment of UK doctors' professionalism: analysis of survey results. BMJ. 2011;343:d6212.

12. Royal College of Physicians London. Revalidation. Available from: http://www.rcplondon.ac.uk/cpd/revalidation. Last accessed Apr 2014.

13. Veloski J, Boex JR, Grasberger MJ, Evans A, Wolfson DB. Systematic review of the literature on assessment, feedback and physicians' clinical performance: BEME Guide No. 7. Med Teach. 2006;28(2):117–28.

14. Dawson D. Fatigue research in 2011: from the bench to practice. Accid Anal Prev. 2012;45(Suppl):1–5.

15. Roach GD, Fletcher A, Dawson D. A model to predict work-related fatigue based on hours of work. Aviat Space Environ Med. 2004;75(3 Suppl):A61–9; discussion A70–4.

16. Fetter RB, Shin Y, Freeman JL, Averill RF, Thompson JD. Case mix definition by diagnosis-related groups. Med Care. 1980;18(2 Suppl):1–53.

17. Doran GT. There's a S.M.A.R.T. way to write managements's goals and objectives. Manage Rev. 1981;70(11):35.

# Chapter 4
## Expertise in Medical Management

**Abstract** Medical managers are uniquely placed combining medical expertise and management skills to allow a deeper understanding of the complex organisation of the health care system. Key amongst the roles of the expert medical manager is the commitment to design and delivery of effective corporate and clinical governance systems.

**Keywords** Problem solving • Local and international health care systems • Corporate and clinical governance systems • Medico-legal aspects of practice • Disaster management response

## Knowledgeable Expert

Medical managers are uniquely placed to bring a clinical background and understanding to bear on the challenges that face health services organisations. Combining medical expertise and management skills allows a deeper understanding of the complex organisation of the health care system in order to produce optimal results for patients, their carers and staff. The health care manager needs wide knowledge of the local, national and international health issues and funding priorities as well as the relevant legislation pertaining to these. In addition she/he will be expected to be familiar with

G. MacCarrick, *Medical Leadership and Management:*
*A Case-based Approach*, DOI 10.1007/978-1-4471-4748-0_4,
© Springer-Verlag London 2014

the advantages and disadvantages of new health technologies, understand the principles of disaster management, be familiar with the medico-legal aspects of clinical practice and be capable of coordinating reviews of health services. Key amongst the roles of the expert medical manager is the commitment to design and delivery of effective corporate and clinical governance systems.

The relevant competencies required of the knowledgeable expert include:

- Demonstrate ability to combine and reconcile medical expertise and management skills in problem solving
- Demonstrate an understanding of best practice in local and international health care systems
- Demonstrate an understanding of relevant legislation pertaining to health care for example privacy, mental health, employment and industrial legislation
- Construct, implement and evaluate effective corporate and clinical governance systems
- Recognise and anticipate relevant medico-legal aspects of practice
- Formulate an appropriate disaster management response plan

## Clinical Governance

Clinical governance is a systematic approach to maintaining and improving the quality of patient care. Defined as "a systematic and integrated approach to assurance and review of clinical responsibility and accountability" [1], its purpose is to optimize patient outcomes. Clinical governance requires health services to assume the same ultimate responsibility for the oversight of the safety and quality of clinical care as they do for financial and business outcomes. The term "integrated governance" has emerged to refer to the combined responsibilities of corporate and clinical governance duties [2].

The need for effective clinical governance in health care has been the subject of significant debate for the past two decades. Since the early 1990s, a number of high profile inquiries and royal commissions have identified significant deficiencies in health care governance systems and processes across the globe. Key inquiries have included Winnipeg Health Sciences Centre (Manitoba Canada) [3], Bristol Royal Infirmary (UK) [4], King Edward Memorial Hospital (WA, Australia) [5], Campbelltown and Camden Hospitals (NSW, Australia) [6] and Bundaberg Base Hospital (Queensland, Australia) [7]. All of these investigations identified a number of underlying themes including the failure of senior management to respond to important safety and quality issues when serious and avoidable adverse events took place in their institutions. In addition typically a culture which did not support open disclosure prevailed. Other contributing factors included poor communication strategies; inadequate credentialing and ineffective clinical and corporate governance.

The economic burden of preventable adverse events is now well documented. In 1992 the first Quality in Australian Health Care Study estimated that adverse events were associated with up to 16.6 % of hospital admissions, subsequently suggesting that nearly half of those events may have been preventable [8]. By 1995 that figure had been revised to 10.6 % [8]. It is now generally accepted that up to 10 % of hospital patients may suffer an adverse event. This is based on the original methodology used in the Harvard Medical Practice Studies [9] and repeated in Australia (1992), New Zealand, United Kingdom and Canada (1998).

The Harvard Medical Practice Study identified that of the hospital admissions associated with adverse errors, 13.6 % led to death and 2.6 % to permanent disability. Drug complications were the most common single type of adverse event (19 %). The Institute of Medicine Committee on Quality of Health Care in America released a report in 1999 *To Err is Human. Building a Safer Health System* [10], estimating that 98,000 Americans die annually due to pre-ventable medical errors, the majority of which are due to system problems rather than poor performance by individuals. The cost of treating adverse events is significant. In one Australian study the total cost of adverse events in their dataset represented an additional 18.6 % of the total inpatient hospital budget [11].

In the United Kingdom the Bristol Royal Infirmary Inquiry (1998) alerted the public to the inadequate standard of care being delivered in paediatric cardiac surgery cases [4]. Included in the nearly 200 recommendations was the need for 'all healthcare professionals' to undergo appraisal, continuing professional development and revalidation to ensure that healthcare professionals remain competent to do their job. Other specific recommendations included in the review were that any unit providing open heart surgery on very young children must have two surgeons trained in paediatric surgery who must undertake a minimum number (between 40 and 50) of open heart operations a year; that the local research ethics committee's permission be sought before any clinician undertakes a new invasive procedure; that doctors must adhere to the principles of open disclosure; that periodic revalidation be compulsory for all healthcare professionals and a national reporting system and database of sentinel events be established.

The main focus of clinical governance is on accountability for care and is based on the principles of high standards of care and transparency. Underpinning clinical governance systems is effective education and training of staff, regular clinical audit, research and clinical risk management. Effective clinical governance requires strong clinical leadership at every level but particularly on the part of the senior medical management.

The effective health care manager must be ever vigilant regarding potential risk. Defined as 'the chance of something happening that will have an impact upon objectives' AS/NZS ISO 31000:2009 [12], risk can impede an organisation's objectives of delivering safe, high quality health care services. Some examples of risk which health care managers are expected to contend with on a regular basis include risks to the availability and quality of patient care, risks to workforce such as the ability to recruit specialist staff, the risk of natural disasters and the risks associated with infection control. Risk management is about putting in place effective processes and structures directed towards managing adverse effects. Integrated risk management is about the systematic application of these processes and structures, both clinical and non-clinical at all levels within the organisation.

Most healthcare managers will be expected to maintain a risk register and oversee risk management processes based on effective communication, risk identification and analysis evaluation and treatment. Managers should be cognisant of an integrated risk management approach when allocating funds, establishing new or modifying existing services and during the management of incidents. Risk management requires regular review and monitoring and is best done using a team-based approach.

The rationale for reporting incidents to improve patient safety is the belief that safety can be improved by learning from incidents and 'near misses'. Investigation of critical incidents was first used in the 1940s by Flanagan [13] as a technique to improve safety and performance among military pilots. Since this time the aviation industry has been used extensively to draw parallels with patient safety. Incident reporting systems in health care should be based on a clear understanding among clinicians about what should be reported and how the reported incidents will be analysed and ultimately lead to changes which will improve patient safety [14]. A useful framework described by Vincent and colleagues [15], has been designed specifically for health care and incorporates elements of Reason's model for organisational accidents [16]. As with other contemporary models of risk management Vincent and Colleagues' model is based on a comprehensive understanding of accident causation, with greater focus on pre-existing organisational factors that provide the conditions in which errors occur [17], rather than merely focusing on the individual who makes the error.

TABLE 4.1 Framework as proposed by Vincent and colleagues [15] for analysing critical incidents in the health sector

| |
| --- |
| **Institutional context**: Economic considerations; regulations; clinical negligence schemes |
| **Organisational and management factors**: Financial resources and constraints; organisational structure; policy standards and goals; safety culture and priorities |
| **Work environment**: Staffing levels and skills mix; workload and shift patterns; design, availability, and maintenance of equipment; administrative and managerial support |
| **Team factors**: Verbal communication; written communication; supervision and seeking help |
| **Team structure**: Individual (staff) factors; knowledge and skills; motivation, physical and mental health |
| **Task factors**: Task design and clarity of structure; availability and use of protocols; availability and accuracy of test results |
| **Patient characteristics**: Condition (complexity and seriousness); language and communication; personality and social factors |

Vincent and colleagues' framework places patients and staff at the first level within the hierarchy, with team factors and working conditions in the middle and institutional factors at the top of the hierarchy (see Table 4.1). Every element of the hierarchy potentially contributes to potential error. The advantage of such a framework is that the emphasis is on examining every level within an organisation, focusing intervention at multiple levels rather than focusing on just one aspect of the organisation. For example in the past a narrow single level approach may have been to enhance staff education to reduce error, ignoring factors such as patient factors, team culture, skill mix or economic constraints [14].

The health care manager has a lead role in planning, implementing, managing and evaluating patient safety initiatives and programs to prevent and address patient harm. A *Clinical Incident* is regarded as any event or circumstance which has actually or could potentially, lead to unintended harm to a patient. Clinical incidents include adverse events, in which harm was actually caused, or Near Miss, in which no harm was caused.

In Australia, the Severity Assessment Code (SAC) matrix assists staff to prioritise and classify incidents and provides a method for quantifying the level of risk associated with an incident by giving the incident a numerical rating (Table 4.2). Management of the incident depends on the level of risk that the incident poses to a patient or patients and/or to the healthcare organisation.

The systematic process for identifying the factors contributing to adverse patient events is referred to as *Root Cause Analysis* (RCA). RCA is simply a determination of what happened, why it happened and how it could be prevented. The organisational level to which an incident must be notified and the timeframe in which this must occur, i.e. the escalation process, is usually specified in each jurisdiction. For example SAC 1 events typically require full escalation whereas SAC 2 & 3 events do not require escalation outside the district or local area network. The medical manager typically plays a significant role in overseeing this process within his/her institution.

## Managing Complaints

Complaints management is a regular part of the health care manager's role and is one mechanism through which adverse events may come to the attention of staff. It is important to recognise that consumer feedback, both positive and negative, is essential in order to provide quality health care services that meet all stakeholder needs. The key principles underpinning an effective complaints management process include accessibility, responsiveness, open disclosure, and accountability. Typically most organisations will have a Complaints Coordinator to facilitate the management of complaints and ensure the complaint management process is efficient and effective.

TABLE 4.2  Severity Assessment Code descriptors used in Queensland Australia [18]

**SAC 1** includes all clinical incidents/near misses where <u>serious harm or death</u> is/could be specifically caused by health care rather than the patient's underlying condition or illness.

**SAC 2** includes all clinical incidents/near misses where <u>moderate harm</u> is/could be specifically caused by health care rather than the patient's underlying condition or illness.

**SAC 3** includes all clinical incidents/near misses where <u>minimal or no harm</u> is/could be specifically caused by health care rather than the patient's underlying condition or illness

**Example Event List (SAC 1)**

Maternal death or serious morbidity associated with labour or delivery

Medication adverse event leading to the death of patient reasonably believed to be due to incorrect management of medications

Intravascular gas embolism resulting in death or neurological damage

Procedures involving the wrong patient or body part resulting in death or likely permanent harm

Retained instruments or other materials after surgery requiring re-operation or further surgical procedure

Haemolytic blood transfusion reaction resulting from ABO incompatibility, resulting in death or likely permanent harm

Suspected suicide of a patient receiving inpatient health care

Complaint management options include resolution at the local level, mediation or referral to another agency. Wherever possible, complaints should be resolved at the point of service delivery in a timely fashion. Most organisations will stipulate compliance with notification timeframes providing time for data collection, investigation, developing an action plan and communicating with relevant parties.

If a clinical incident has occurred that results in harm to a patient while receiving health care then *open disclosure* should take place [18]. Open Disclosure generally has two aspects. Clinician open disclosure is the informal process where the treating clinician informs the patient that an incident has occurred, expressing regret for the harm caused or adverse outcome, whereas formal open disclosure, is the structured process to ensure communication between the patient and/or family, senior clinicians and the organisation. Key elements of the process include a factual explanation to the patient as to what occurred and the potential consequences as well as the steps being taken to manage the event and prevent recurrence.

## Managing Disasters

Disaster Response Management is a feature of the health care manager's expert role. An emergency is an actual or imminent event which endangers life and/or property requiring a coordinated response. A disaster is a serious disruption to community life which exceeds the usual capacity of local resources and which requires a significant coordinated response to help the community recover from the disruption. A serious disruption is typically defined as: (a) loss of human life or illness or injury to humans, (b) widespread or severe property loss or damage and/or (c) widespread or severe damage to the environment. The key elements of disaster emergency response are preparedness, prevention, response and recovery [19, 20]. In terms of preparedness, once a hazard analysis of the local community has been undertaken arrangements can be put in place to deal with future potential threats according to the following principles:

1. Organisation: Disaster response Management needs to be supported by an organisational structure so that future responsibilities for prevention, preparedness, response and recovery can be established.
2. Command and control: It must be clear to all involved in a disaster who is in control and what the organisational command structure within each agency is. This is typically specified in legislation and in the local disaster plan.

3. Coordination and support: The disaster plan will stipulate the authority and responsibility for assembling resources which are required.
4. Information Management: Appropriate communication networks need to be established in advance.
5. Timely activation: Activation of the disaster plan should take place in a timely fashion.
6. An effective disaster plan

Once an emergency is realised the duty medical director typically assesses the situation, determines if it is a disaster, notifies his/her chain of command and media officer, consults the State emergency plan and alerts key contact officers. If the situation meets the definition of a disaster then he/she establishes the emergency operating centre, (EOC). The EOC is the control facility responsible for carrying out the principles of emergency or disaster management. The EOC should be of adequate size, location and access – typically encompassing a debriefing room conference room and sufficient amenities including catering and parking. The facility also requires sufficient supplies such as telecommunications, IT support and consumables.

Following every disaster response plan is a period of recovery management, which must also be planned for. A number of concepts provide the basis for effective recovery management and these include: community involvement; management at the local level; a community-based approach; empowering individuals and communities; planned and timely withdrawal; flexibility adaptability and responsiveness; and coordination and integration of services including appropriate resourcing arrangements. Experience has shown that the recovery phase is most effective when individuals and communities actively participate in the management of their own recovery.

In summary, medical managers must possess a defined body of expert knowledge, skills, and professional attitudes, which are directed to ensuring the delivery of effective and safe patient care. The manager applies these competencies to collect and interpret information, analyse and synthesise investigations and make appropriate decisions. This is done in partnership with patients, other health care providers and the community. As the scope of the manager's expertise is broad, ranging from oversight of clinical governance to disaster response management, the manager also needs to recognize the limits of their own expertise, knowing when to seek appropriate advice from other health professionals.

## Case Study 1

You are the Director of Medical Services for a 200 bed regional hospital. There are several Visiting orthopedic surgeons and one full time staff specialist Orthopedic surgeon. The staff specialist is very close to retirement. He comes to see you to report a higher than normal rate of post – operative infection following elective hip replacements. Most of the hip replacements at the hospital are done by the four visiting surgeons who attend different theatres on different days. The staff specialist comes to you and says that the standard of care by the surgeons is "going downhill" and there are too many post-operative infections. He also adds that "this is what you can expect with the new policy of employing part-time visiting staff (at the expense of full time staff specialists)" who have "no loyalty to the hospital and are not concerned with participating in Quality Improvement activities of the Department".

You later happen to meet the hospital Patient Safety Officer in the corridor who reports she has not noticed any increase in infection rates recently but would look in to it for you and provide a report at the next Infection Control meeting.

Later that day you receive a phone call from the Patient Complaints officer, who advises that a prominent member of the community (the local MP), has undergone a recent hip replacement and suffered a "nasty post-operative infection". She thought she should let you know as the family were most distressed and in case there was any further action.

**What additional information will you seek?**
**How will you manage this situation?**
Consider:

- Individual and collective patient safety. What is the current clinical governance practice and how is post-operative infection recorded and audited?
- Specifically, what arrangements for monitoring clinical outcomes are currently in place and do these extend to Visiting staff?
- Is this a real problem? What evidence is available for the Staff specialist surgeon's claims?
- How you will investigate, assess and manage clinical performance of visiting and full–time staff?
- How is the current patient complaint being managed? Has appropriate support and follow up been arranged?
- Review patient's file and ensure appropriate open disclosure.
- Ensure clinical incident is recorded and arrangements in place for appropriate clinical incident review.
- Establish if disparity exists between staff specialist assessment of post operate complication and reported cases of infection.
- If inadequate or under-reporting of clinical incidents by staff then why? Consider conducting a full chart audit if concerns are serious.
- If outcomes are indeed poor and do not meet a minimum standard of care (based on benchmarking and review of the literature) then consider solutions such as, training, protocol review, limiting the scope of practice through credentialing and regular clinical audit.

## Case Study 2

You are the newly appointed director of medical services for a regional hospital. Each Friday you attend grand rounds as you enjoy staying in touch with the clinical cases of interest to your training specialists. Following grand rounds you have the opportunity to spend lunch with consultants and training doctors as well as medical students. You overhear a conversation between two medical students regarding one of your obstetricians performing a potential hysterectomy on the 15-year-old girl with significant intellectual disability. It appears one of the medical students plans to discuss the case at a forthcoming ethics seminar later that week. When you get back to the office, you speak with the director of nursing who confirms that Dr X routinely performs ster-ilisation procedures in cases such as this in your hospital. The director of nursing is aware of this scheduled case for tomorrow as one of her own nurses has expressed her own concerns and even raised the possibility with the Director of Nursing (DON) of going to the media. You contact Dr X and arrange a meeting. He has been a staff member at the hospital for 15 years. He seems taken aback at your concerns which include the legal implications of perform-ing a procedure even if the parents have consented. He reluctantly agrees to defer the procedure until you have investigated further, but insists you explain your decision to the family.

**What are the key issues here?**
**How will you manage these?**

- Seek immediate legal advice.
- Source relevant legislation relating to guardianship, family law and any relevant Court rulings.
- Considerate prohibiting the procedure until full advice has been obtained.
- Notify other consultants of the interim decision
- Arrange to speak to the patient and her parents and explain decision.
- Have other contraceptive options been considered?
- Plan time to discuss with Dr X. How does he obtain informed consent?
- How does Dr X minimise risk (including anaesthetic risk) in situations such as this?
- Have there been previous complaints?
- Anticipate potential media involvement and their management

## Case Study 3

You are the Acting CEO of the local hospital. On your way home for the long weekend at to your holiday home on the Coast you hear over the radio that an inbound flight has reported an issue and possible engine failure en route to your regional airport. The pilot has issued a Mayday and emergency services are gathering at the airport awaiting the arrival of the flight carrying 100 passengers. Most of the passengers are tourists from overseas, many non-English speaking.

It has been 2 years since you have conducted a desktop exercise with the local airport and you are aware that significant senior staff changes have taken place at the airport and in the local State Emergency Services in the interim.

**What are your immediate priorities/concerns?**
**What will you consider in the long term?**
Consider the following:

- Activate emergency services
- Alert the health Department and minister's office notify media officer
- establish EOC, Links with Ambulance, Police, Fire services – how to include those people and establishing chain of command on site
- hazards, actual and potential
- access and egress
- numbers of people involved
- translation services
- emergency services at the site or required
- Principles of triage
- Crowd control (passengers and people waiting for them)
- Mobilisation of resources after hours and long weekend
- Counselling for passengers and staff involved
- Divert other inbound flights
- Media and political issues
- Communication issues in a disaster –secure phone lines
- Placing hospital and others in the region on standby
- triage in multi casualty disaster

- Recovery phase
- when briefing others consider 'TSMEAC', i.e.

  - **T**opography – consider maps, sketches, models.
  - **S**ituation – consider a general description of what has taken place in the details, exact location
  - **M**ission – generate a clear and concise statement of the purpose of the organisation's involvement
  - **E**xecution – generate a general outline describing how it is intended to carry out the mission, detailing any particular phases and indicating groups if any to be deployed.
  - **A**dministration and logistics -for example medical, equipment, catering, stores, transport, accommodation and evacuation instructions.
  - **C**ommand and communications – consider a location of command posts and identification of key position holders for example communication controllers etc.

# References

1. Department of Health of Western Australia. Clinical governance, the framework of assurance, Department of Health of WA, 2001. 2001. Available from: http://www.safetyandquality. health.wa.gov.au/docs/clinical_gov/Executive_Summary_Paper. pdf. Cited Apr 2014.
2. Beech R, Henderson C, Ashby S, Dickinson A, Sheaff R, Windle K, Wistow G, Knapp M. Does integrated governance lead to integrated patient care? Findings from the innovation forum. Health Soc Care Community. 2013;21(6):598–605.
3. Davies JM. Painful inquiries: lessons from Winnipeg. Can Med Assoc J. 2001;165(11):1503–4.
4. The Bristol Royal Infirmary Inquiry. Learning from Bristol: the report of the public inquiry into children's heart surgery at the Bristol Royal Infirmary 1984–1995. 2001. Available from: http:// urlm.co.uk/www.bristol-inquiry.org.uk.
5. Western Australia. Inquiry into Obstetric Gynaecological Services at King Edward Memorial Hospital, Douglas N, editors. Inquiry into obstetric and gynaecological services at King Edward Memorial Hospital, 1990–2000: final report. Perth: The Inquiry; 2001.

6. Walker B. Interim report of the Special Commission of Inquiry into Campbelltown and Camden Hospitals. In: Walker, B. (ed.) Pandora electronic collection. 2004. [Accessed from http://nla.gov.au/nla.cat-vn3123549.

7. Queensland Public Hospitals Commission of Inquiry. 2005. Available from: http://www.health.qld.gov.au/inquiry/.

8. Wilson RM, Harrison BT, Gibberd RW, Hamilton JD. An analysis of the causes of adverse events from the Quality in Australian Health Care Study. Med J Aust. 1999;170(9):411–5.

9. Brennan TA, Leape LL, Laird NM, Hebert L, Localio AR, Lawthers AG, Newhouse JP, Weiler PC, Hiatt HH. Incidence of adverse events and negligence in hospitalized patients. Results of the Harvard Medical Practice Study I. N Engl J Med. 1991;324(6):370–6.

10. Donaldson MS, Kohn LT, Corrigan J. To err is human: building a safer health system. Washington, DC: The National Academies Press; 2000.

11. Ehsani JP, Jackson T, Duckett SJ. The incidence and cost of adverse events in Victorian hospitals 2003–04. Med J Aust. 2006;184(11):551–5.

12. International Organization for Standardization. ISO 31000 – Risk management. Available from: http://www.iso.org/iso/home/standards/iso31000.htm. Cited Apr 2014.

13. Flanagan JC. The critical incident technique. Psychol Bull. 1954;51(4):327–58.

14. Mahajan RP. Critical incident reporting and learning. Br J Anaesth. 2010;105(1):69–75.

15. Vincent C, Taylor-Adams S, Stanhope N. Framework for analysing risk and safety in clinical medicine. BMJ. 1998;316(7138):1154–7.

16. Reason JT. Human error. Cambridge, UK: Cambridge University Press; 1990.

17. Vincent C. Clinical risk management: enhancing patient safety 2001. 2nd ed. London: BMJ Books; 2001.

18. Australian Commission on Safety and Quality in Health Care, editor. Australian open disclosure framework. Sydney: Australian Commission on Safety and Quality in Health Care; 2013.

19. Born CT, Briggs SM, Ciraulo DL, Frykberg ER, Hammond JS, Hirshberg A, Lhowe DW, O'Neill PA. Disasters and mass casualties: I. General principles of response and management. J Am Acad Orthop Surg. 2007;15(7):388–96.

20. O'Neill PA. The ABC's of disaster response. Scand J Surg. 2005;94(4):259–66.

# Chapter 5
## The Adaptable Communicator

**Abstract** The ability to communicate effectively with diverse groups is a necessary part of the medical manager's role. The adaptable communicator will consider the message and how it is presented to diverse audiences in different contexts. In addition the effective communicator should demonstrate active listening skills.

**Keywords** Communication with diverse groups • Interpersonal communication • Teaching • Media management

## Adaptable Communicator

The ability to communicate effectively in different settings and with diverse groups is a necessary part of the medical manager's role. Effective communication is an essential part of achieving individual and organizational goals. One of the most cited models of communication is that of Shannon and Weaver [1]. Most models describe five components to the communication process; – the communicator; the message; the medium; the receiver and feedback. The effective leader will recognize these elements and be able to identify blocks to communication as well as identifying strategies to improve interpersonal communication. Within most organizations, communication travels in three main directions, upward downward and horizontally. The adaptable communicator will manage flow of communication in all directions on a daily basis, and will be cognizant of regulating the flow of information and providing regular feedback. In addition the effective manager will consider the message and how it is presented to different audiences and demonstrate active listening skills.

The relevant competencies required of an adaptable communicator include:

- Understands the components of the communication process
- Identifies blocks to the sending and receiving of information
- Demonstrated ability to engage with stakeholders internal and external to the organisation
- Ability to convey relevant information and explanations to diverse groups
- Understands strategies for improving interpersonal communication
- Understands the purpose of various effective communication methodologies and chooses the most appropriate in a given situation
- Demonstrated role as teacher
- Demonstrates appropriate use of the media

Medical managers engage with a variety of stakeholders every day and regularly communicate across the health care organization. The ability to tailor the message to different stakeholders and adapt communication styles for different stakeholders is key. The unique position occupied by the medical manager is the ability to convey both the clinical and management perspectives. Often health care requires understanding of complex issues. Analysis and synthesis of information is required in the formulation of policy and the medical manager regularly relies on the ability to communicate complex expert knowledge to a variety of stakeholders.

Addressing confusion, misunderstanding and even hostility [2–4] as well as delivering bad news [5] are some of the key challenges in medicine. These skills also apply to the medical manager. Before delivering bad news it is worth considering the potential reaction of the recipient which at times can be unpredictable. For instance in some situations the receipt of bad news may come with a sense of relief and in some situations good news can be perceived as distressing. It is also important to consider who is best placed to deliver bad news as well as the timing and place of delivery. Empathy coupled with active listening skills are paramount [6].

A particular communication challenge for the medical manager is the obtaining of *consent* and the assessment of competence to give consent before a medical procedure is carried out. Key to the obtaining of informed consent is the need to ensure the patient fully understands the procedure to be carried out and the potential side effects. It is often useful to ascertain what the person already knows before providing additional information and to clarify with the patient their understanding after the exchange of information. A useful technique is to ask the patient to summarise what was agreed or what was communicated. The medical manager needs to understand the importance of imparting knowledge using different techniques such as in writing, verbally, with the use of visual aids or indeed using translator services.

## Writing a Business Case

One of the key practical communication skills required of the medical manager is the ability to write a *business case*. Such a submission is often required to initiate a new plan or for approval for the development or expansion of existing resources. A business case will typically contain an analysis of costs and benefits associated with any proposed initiative or development and will identify various other options for delivery such as expansion of an existing service or outsourcing. A project plan will often accompany a business case and will list project objectives, outcomes, scope and timeframe. A Gantt chart (Fig. 5.1) is often a useful appendix. The business case

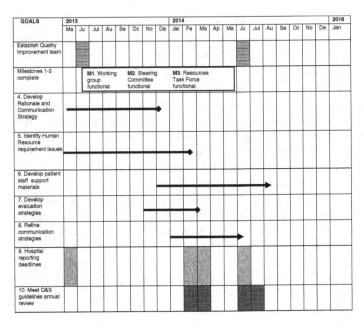

FIGURE 5.1  The Gannt chart included in this editor's proof is incomplete. A complete Gannt chart is attached as a separate file

will often make reference to specific project management strategies, proposed milestones and expected timeframes, required resources and training; communication strategies, relevant policy or legislation and proposed plans for quality assurance.

The submission should clearly describe how the benefits of the proposal will be evaluated for each of the alternatives. If the project is expected to have operational impact, (for example on equipment, administration, information technology) then this should also be included. Likewise if the project is expected to have clinical impact (for example on the number of surgical lists per week, emergency department waiting times) then there should be a plan to capture this activity data.

When preparing a business case it is important to clearly identify time specific and measurable project outcomes. Where possible it is often helpful to justify the business case with supporting data such as activity trends and indicators. If the business case required consultation with stakeholders then this should be reported. Any additional services required to implement the new initiative should also be included for example allied health support. The submission should also include recurrent and non-recurrent costs such as establishment costs, ongoing maintenance costs and human resource requirements. As with any project plan it is best practice to include a risk management outline, identifying risks associated with both implementing and not implementing the proposed change. The proposal should articulate the scope or boundaries of the proposed project and any inclusion or exclusion criteria as well as the proposed governance structure.

## Teaching

Teaching peers and juniors is a particularly important aspect of the medical manger's role as communicator. Medical managers will typically be involved in support of a variety of educational programs for junior and senior doctors such as local medical education units [7], post-graduate education and supervision and specialist training post accreditation as well as generic education and training such as computer and management skills; clinical skills sessions (including Grand rounds, morbidity/mortality review sessions) and skills development centres. Apart from the support of teaching, medical managers should be skilled as teachers themselves. By modelling personal educational strategies such as self-directed learning, managers provide powerful examples for their trainees to follow. They can also assist trainees in facilitating self-direction in learning through assistance with goal setting and feedback. Managers should also teach in a manner which recognizes the different educational needs of different learner groups, as well as the different learning style [8, 9]. Effective clinical teachers are those that act as role models and are also supportive supervisors [10]. It stands to reason that the same can be said of medical managers who teach and supervise trainees in the discipline of medical management and leadership. A number of bed-side teaching competency frameworks have been described [11, 12] which can be adapted to the management setting (See Chap. 8).

## Delivering an Oral Presentation

Apart from teaching there are many other occasions when the medical director is required to deliver an oral presentation to colleagues or other stakeholders as part of their executive role. Oral presentations are regularly made at meetings, conferences and forums. A useful way to commence is to have a well-constructed session plan which includes the aims and objectives of the session, the resources required to deliver the session, timing, strategies to be used and evaluation strategies. The strategies included in any presentation will depend on the purpose of the presentation and the audience and can include demonstrations, simulations, role plays or group discussion. If the presentation has an educational focus then it is good practice to begin with a set of learning objectives, phrased in such a way as to allow the presenter and the audience to measure that learning has taken place. When writing learning objectives it is necessary to be clear, concise and concrete. There are several texts available to assist in the writing of well-constructed learning objectives [13]. A consideration of required resources will include availability of site e.g. video players, OHPs, slide projector or whiteboard and even whiteboard markers, spare pens or spare OHP bulbs. Any technical considerations such as compatibility issues related to use of computers will need to be dealt with in advance. A consideration of timing issues will include start and finish times, proposed break times, timing of different parts of the session and sufficient allocated times for inclusion of video clips etc.

In general presentations tend to be successful if there is personal motivation to understand the concepts, if the material presented is relevant and important and pitched at an appropriate level and if there is active involvement by the audience. Producing a structured presentation that is logical and coherent is critical. It is often useful to begin by creating an introduction that clearly states the purpose of the presentation. If the purpose is to provide an explanation (for example the rationale for a decision made by hospital executive) then ensuring that the introduction includes a clear statement of the question or problem and an outline of how you propose to address it is helpful. Keeping to the point and avoiding digression or inclusion of irrelevant material is key. As much as possible it is important to construct a presentation that consists of a logical argument with a sound conclusion supported by valid and relevant evidence. It is often helpful to audiences to highlight the key points in the material as the presentation is being delivered and re-emphasising these points in the conclusion.

The choice of language will depend on the audience. For example a presentation to peers will be expected to contain discipline specific vocabulary whereas a presentation to a lay group will be expected to be free of jargon. Most presentations typically use variety of media and if a slide presentation is chosen then it will be important to select material for slides that is directly relevant to the task that the presentation is intended to address. Correct referencing of any images employed and any quotations or data from the work of others needs to be acknowledged and is a particular professional consideration.

Simple strategies such as using a font in the projected images large enough for the audience to be able to read clearly including sizing images of all diagrams, tables, data and the like to be clear and readable from all parts of the room, is always an important factor to consider. As a rule it is important to avoid too many words in the projected image as it can contribute to confusion or boredom. An alternative is to include printed handouts, where there is an excessive amount of data or number of words to transmit to the audience.

Finally any presentation should include some form of evaluation. This might include a formal written evaluation form administered after the presentation asking the audience to comment on how well the learning objectives were met.

## Chairing Meetings

Meetings are a regular feature of the working life of medical managers. They are a group process and as such require an understanding of group dynamics. Effective meetings require effective chairs in order to achieve their aims. The following tips may be helpful in chairing successful meetings.

Prior to the meeting, it is worth challenging the necessity of the meeting in the first place. It is worth considering whether a more effective means of communicating is available that might obviate the need to gather busy people together particularly in complex organisations such as hospitals and health services. In advance it is also worth articulating clearly the objectives of the meeting and what is to be achieved. Having in mind potential the anticipated outcome of the meeting including the best potential result and the minimum acceptable result is a useful consideration. Not only is the chairing of the meeting important but also the membership:

> Both the chair and membership confer power that can be very influential, particularly when resources are being allocated. There is said to be only one thing worse hat being a member of a committee and that is not to be a member (p 87.) [14]

It is always necessary to review and research the agenda or issues and consider who can provide the best expertise when defining the membership. In advance itemise agenda items and timeframes and ensure all stakeholders have been notified in a timely manner of the agenda.

During the meeting, it is useful to begin with introductions and providing an overview of the meetings objectives. As chair it is important to keep meeting focused with good time keeping. Directing discussion towards the stipulated meeting aims and utilising membership expertise whilst ensuring everyone feels heard are also important. If a particular issue arises which was not anticipated but which dominates the agenda, then it may need to be deferred to a dedicated meeting. Encourage constructive discussion and debate throughout whilst at the same time maintaining a professional code of order, ensuring only one person speaks at a time. At the end of the meeting it is important to summarise in a timely manner before the membership disperses. Everyone should be clear what took place and understands actions which are required, by whom and by when. After the meeting is concluded timely distribution of minutes should occur. It is a useful exercise to evaluate meetings with the membership to ensure they are continuing to meet the agreed objectives and identify any potential future improvements in terms of conduct, chairing, membership etc.

## Media Management

The public media is another fundamental communication tool with which the manager will be expected to be familiar. As a medical manager it is important to have an understanding of how to engage with and use the media appropriately and effectively. Contentious issues which are likely to generate strong or prolonged media interest or debate are typically directed to the local director of the media unit. Most hospitals will have a unit responsible for media and corporate communications. Nonetheless, requests for local media releases often end up on the medical manager's desk and the media office can assist with the preparation of the release, including briefing the spokesperson and preparing for a media interview. Managing the media during a medical emergency or disaster is a particular function often filled by a senior medical manager. Typically this involves liaison with external agencies such as Police and Emergency Services.

It is important to be aware of the legal aspects of media use. For example patients have a right to interact with the media and a right to be informed of any requests for media interaction. This includes the right to allow detailed information of a personal nature to be released publicly. In terms of release of patient information however, the medical manager needs to be aware of the duty-of-confidentiality obligations which apply to all patients as well as the relevant legislation regarding release of information and guidelines for handling patient information, such as codes of conduct and Privacy Acts. In most situations written consent must be obtained from the patient or their legal guardian.

When asked to provide general information regarding a patient's condition (and with consent), the typical descriptors used are:

- **good condition**: vital signs are stable and within normal limits; patient is conscious and comfortable; indicators are excellent
- **stable**: vital signs are stable and within normal limits; patient is conscious but may not be comfortable; indicators are favourable
- **serious**: vital signs may be unstable and not within normal limits; patient is acutely ill; indicators are questionable
- **critical**: vital signs are unstable and not within normal limits; patient may not be conscious; indicators are unfavourable

Media interviews are often requested from senior medical staff. It is important to recognise that staff have no obligation to participate in any media arrangements, if they chose not to. If an interview is to be given it is often helpful to practise delivering the key message in advance. Repeating the key messages throughout the interview, using plain language and avoidance of jargon or technical terms will help deliver a simple message. It is important to stay calm and speak clearly and succinctly and listen carefully to questions and clarify any question you don't understand as anything said will remain on record. Avoiding commenting on issues outside one's area of expertise and avoiding commentary on political matters or government policy issues as well as any matters related to future government funding is good practice. As a rule news interviews will be short with the journalist looking for a short "voice grab" whereas talkbacks/current affairs interviews will be longer. It is important to prepare well in advance for the topic and have accurate and up to date facts and statistics written or available.

In summary medical managers facilitate effective communication through shared decision-making and effective and dynamic interactions with a myriad of stakeholders including colleagues, patients, families, funding bodies and other stakeholders. Communication skills, considered essential in the therapeutic relationship for establishing rapport and trust and delivering information on formulated diagnoses are also relevant to the medical manager. The medical manager seeks to achieve mutual understanding between an increasing number of stakeholders in a progressively more complex environment of health care delivery. Accurately eliciting and synthesizing information and conveying relevant information to stakeholders to achieve shared understanding on issues, using a wide variety of media are competencies critical to the medical manager's role.

## Case Study 1

You are the established Medical Director of a public teaching hospital and one of your senior clinicians (a pathologist) comes to see you about concerns she has about clinical outcomes at the affiliated private hospital. For some years now your hospital has relied on the next door private hospital to conduct gynaecological oncology services. Recently you were introduced to the new gynaecological oncologist and you recall how excited he was about the possibilities his new appointment would provide for patients of both hospitals. Your pathologist is concerned that she has reviewed the outcomes of the surgery being conducted and according to her own analysis, the outcomes over the past 6 months have been significantly poorer than expected especially when compared with the previous oncologist. Your pathologist tells you she had brought these results to the attention of her Head of Department who appeared to do nothing with the data. She then advises that she went a further step to share the results with the previous oncologist now retired but editor of the local medical association journal. It is also widely known that he was not too pleased about his successor's appointment - concerned he was too young to take on his established practice.

The now retired oncologist has emailed your pathologist indicating he intends (with her permission) to take her report to the media.

**What are the main issues and how will you prioritise and manage these?**

- Make time to prioritise this matter as patients are continuing to be referred
- Establish the facts
- What is the significance of the Pathologist Report?
- Consider ceasing referrals pending your investigation? Foremost is your duty of care to patients
- Consider how to manage this episode of 'whistle blowing' and how to build relationship with the pathologist. How to manage whistle blowing more generally in the organisation
- Do you have established communication lines with the retired oncologist? If so can you exploit this established relationship and explore concerns/perceptions
- Are there any other relevant background factors to the complaint?
- Why has the HOD not acted upon it? Was the analysis statistically sound/flawed?
- Consider relationship with the neighbouring hospital and lines of communication with them over morbidity/mortality data
- May need to consider selecting an expert panel considering membership, terms of reference and feedback to you
- Consider compare outcomes with national and international benchmarks
- Media management, assume the report has been leaked and anticipate outcome
- Manage the communication process with CEO and Board of Management

# Case Study 2

You are a director of medical services for a regional hospital. The local population is growing rapidly owing to an increased number of retirees moving into the area. As each year passes the hospital is under increasing pressure and several of the service areas have already outstripped the hospital's ability to support them. With a local endocrinologist having retired the diabetes service is under critical pressure. At a recent conference you have become aware of the concept of Hospital in the Home (HITH). Using this model some hospitals have been able to select particular types of health care which can be delivered more effectively in the home. You are also aware that diabetes services can be provided this way. You decide to convince your CEO that this is a worthwhile undertaking.

**How would you convince the CEO and the board that this new innovation is worthwhile considering?**

**What are the issues involved and how would you overcome them?**

- Prepare a business case articulating the current financial pressures on the hospital and the cost effectiveness of alternative models including Hospital in the home
- articulate the key issues
- analyse the current service delivery
- discuss plans for a stakeholder consultation
- includes outcomes from other centres using Hospital in the Home
- provide a systematic analysis of alternatives setting out criteria to help members of the board choose amongst the options available
- cost the alternatives
- define an action plan including budgets project schedules, Gantt charts and regulatory measures including evaluation
- describe potential range of services that could be provided
- articulate potential goals and milestones
- define population, staff requirements, waiting times etc.
- discuss benchmarking to compare outputs with other centres

- describe communication strategy
- discuss all of the above with reference to safety, effectiveness, appropriateness, efficiency, access and consumer group participation

# References

1. Shannon CE, Weaver W. The mathematical theory of communication. Urbana: University of Illinois Press; 1964.
2. Scott T. Sudden traumatic death: caring for the bereaved. Trauma. 2007;9(2):103–9.
3. Parris RJ. Initial management of bereaved relatives following trauma. Trauma. 2012;14(2):139–55.
4. Klein S, Alexander DA. Good grief: a medical challenge. Trauma. 2003;5(4):261–71.
5. Maguire P, Faulkner A. Communicate with cancer patients: 1. Handling bad news and difficult questions. BMJ. 1988;297(6653): 907–9.
6. Pendleton D. The new consultation: developing doctor-patient communication. Oxford/New York: Oxford University Press; 2003.
7. Davis MH, Karunathilake I, Harden RM. AMEE Education Guide no. 28: the development and role of departments of medical education. Med Teach. 2005;27(8):665–75.
8. Chapman DM, Calhoun JG. Validation of learning style measures: implications for medical education practice. Med Educ. 2006;40(6):576–83.
9. Smits PBA, Verbeek JHAM, Nauta MCE, Ten Cate TJ, Metz JCM, Van Dijk FJH. Factors predictive of successful learning in postgraduate medical education. Med Educ. 2004;38(7):758–66.
10. Irby DM, Ramsey PG, Gillmore GM, Schaad D. Characteristics of effective clinical teachers of ambulatory care medicine. Acad Med. 1991;66(1):54–5.
11. Lake FR. Teaching on the run tips: doctors as teachers. Med J Aust. 2004;180(8):415–6.
12. Lake FR, Vickery AW. Teaching on the run tips 14: teaching in ambulatory care. Med J Aust. 2006;185(3):166–7.
13. Kennedy D. Writing and using learning outcomes – a practical guide. Ireland: University College Cork; 2007.
14. Lawson JS, Rotem A, O'Rourke I, Forde K, Bates P. From clinician to manager: an introduction to hospital and health service management. 2nd ed. Sydney: McGraw-Hill; 2004. xii, 236 p.

# Chapter 6
## The Creative Collaborator

**Abstract** Medical managers build effective relationships with a myriad of stakeholders including other colleagues, patients, their families and carers, funders and policy makers to achieve improvement in health outcomes.

**Keywords** Building and maintaining effective relationships • Inter-professional healthcare teams • Conflict resolution • Construction and management of teams

## Creative Collaborator

As medical managers and leaders health care professionals must be able to build effective relationships with a myriad of stakeholders including other colleagues, patients, their families and carers, funders and policy makers to achieve improvement in health outcomes. The medical manager should be able to participate in and lead inter-professional healthcare teams, displaying a positive attitude to team members and effectively work with other health professionals to prevent, negotiate and resolve conflict. Whenever it is necessary to form new groups, the medical manager must be able to construct teams with appropriate membership, recognizing the principles of group behavior and effectively pursuing the expert contribution of each key member.

G. MacCarrick, *Medical Leadership and Management:*
*A Case-based Approach*, DOI 10.1007/978-1-4471-4748-0_6,
© Springer-Verlag London 2014

> The relevant competencies of the creative collaborator in medical management include:
>
> - Develop, build and maintain effective relationships with all stakeholders, forming constructive alliances
> - Participate in and lead inter-professional healthcare teams
> - Negotiate and resolve conflict
> - Understanding of construction and management of teams
> - Demonstrates the principles of relational leadership as a collaborative social process
> - Demonstrates the ability to entertain multiple perspectives

Medical managers engage in and facilitate consultation on a daily basis. It is important to maintain at all times a respectful attitude towards colleagues and members of the inter-professional team to prevent and resolve any conflict. As part of this the manager is expected to respect individual differences and understand the relevant politics. Excellent conflict management and high level communication, negotiation and interpersonal skills are mandatory.

In most situations it is necessary to make decisions when faced with multiple and conflicting perspectives. To do so it is necessary to be able to use a variety of mechanisms for consultative purposes and cope with complex and uncertain situations. Building and maintaining effective constructive alliances is key. Understanding and respecting group dynamics, including professional boundaries and bureaucracy, is a necessary part of problem solving in the complex health care setting.

The exercise of leadership and management in professional bureaucracies such as health care is challenging. Medical managers are faced with the task of leading clinical colleagues who are often motivated by allegiance to their respective professional bodies rather than their host organizations. Increasingly healthcare management is conceptualized as a collaborative social process, evidenced by relationship building [1].

# Relational Leadership

*Relational leadership* is an adaptive and iterative process of engagement between people in organisations [2, 3]. Relational leaders require an understanding of how individuals in an organization make sense of their lived experience i.e. 'sense-making' [4]. Sense making is an important concept in healthcare where the ability to entertain multiple perspectives is a particular challenge. In health care, effective leadership is often evidenced by the brokerage of relationships between stakeholder groups, achieved through influence, building relationships trust and respect and inspiring the actions of others [1]. The relational approach also requires a deep interest in the narratives of others, i.e. how others narrate their lived experience through storytelling [5, 6]. Storytelling is not new in either the discipline of medicine or organizational behavior. Descriptive narrative research has an established place in describing change in organizations and has been used by organizational analysts to help understand how we make sense of events in our lives and within organizations [5, 7, 8]. Thomas and Znaniecki, authors of the landmark life history *The Polish Peasant,* pointed to the value of narrative in the context of organizations [9]:

> A social institution can be fully understood only if we do not limit ourselves to the abstract study of its formal organization, but analyze the way in which it appears in the personal experience of various members of the group and follow the influence which it has upon their lives [9] (p. 1833).

Polkinghorne [10] describes the place of narrative in our daily lives as follows:

> Our lives are ceaselessly intertwined with narrative, with the stories that we tell and hear told, with the stories that we dream or imagine or would like to tell. All these stories are reworked in that story of our own lives which we narrate to ourselves in an episodic, sometimes semiconscious, virtually uninterrupted monologue (p. 160)

Boje [11] describes storytelling in organizations as the "preferred sense-making currency of human relationships", forming part of an information-processing network [11] (p. 106). The use of narrative research by organizational analysts has helped uncover the "values" and "assumptions" of an organization. Listening carefully to the stories of colleagues and co-workers the medical manager can ascertain whether the members of the organization hold to a single story as part of what Polkinghorne refers to as "a coherent organizational narrative" (p. 162) or whether there are multiple narratives within the same organization. Listening to the stories and accounts of co –workers can also inform the medical manager and alert him/her to the possibility of conflict, particularly between different groups or between individuals.

## Managing Conflict

Conflict in the workplace can result in reduced productivity, staff dissatisfaction, and a negative work environment. The traditional view of conflict is that it is deleterious and must be prevented. A more contemporary view sees conflict as sometimes necessary and an inevitable part of the group process. Some conflict is seen as necessary and in fact each organization has a particular optimal level of conflict. Dysfunctional conflict is that which exceeds the optimal level and has potential to harm the organization [12]. It is useful for the medical manager to be able to gauge the level of conflict within his/her organization. Several models of conflict have been described which define the cause, impact and consequences of conflict. Pondy's earliest model described stages of latency, feeling, perception, manifestation, and aftermath [13]. The medical manager needs to be familiar with these stages as conflict can be more difficult to manage as it progresses through these stages. Conflict can occur within and between different health care groups and can result in negative stereotyping and decreased communication. The primary focus of the manager therefore should be to resolve conflict situations promptly before they escalate. Some simple strategies to employ when bringing parties together to discuss their issues include choosing an appropriate time to bring conflicting parties together to discuss. Plan in advance what you are going to say and stick to the facts. During the meeting avoid apportioning blame and allow each party to express their point of view. Active listening through paraphrasing to ensure you and the others convey meaning and understanding. As a facilitator it is imperative to maintain objectivity and direct meetings away from destructive confrontation towards constructive understanding and resolution. It is also important that suggested solutions are in fact feasible and if so that the parties commit to their implementation. It is often useful to establish some form of follow up at a later stage to meet and discuss how things are progressing. Where possible, grievance resolution should be attempted at the local level, however, in some situations it may not be possible to achieve resolution and an alternate dispute resolution approach may be required. Formal grievance resolution is typically managed by the local Human Resource Management Unit. Whichever means is used, the process should be fair, transparent and timely.

The medical manager should be familiar with local policies relating to grievance procedures, allegations of sexual harassment or racial discrimination, disciplinary procedures, fraud, criminal or official misconduct, patient complaints and workplace equity.

## Inter-professional Care

Team work and inter-professional care [14] are becoming more central to health care as more evidence emerges that effective teamwork directly enhances the quality of patient care. There are increasing demands for effective professional partnerships, particularly as health systems adapt to caring for patients that require long term management of chronic disease. The focus is increasingly towards health care that is holistic in nature [15]. The medical manager's role as leader of inter-professional teams is to encourage the contribution of all team members, displaying a positive attitude and integrating the contributions of all members. In 2001 the Institute of Medicine published the report *Crossing the Quality Chasm: A New Health System for the 21st Century.* This report [16] concluded that a major overhaul of the health care system was required and stressed that such a redesigned system should be predicated on multidisciplinary teams. Several other reports have since advocated the same redesign. One of the key challenges in embedding inter-professional care is creating the opportunity to learn together at an undergraduate level. It is unrealistic to expect health care providers to work together in teams when they have not been educated together, nor continue to learn together to develop team-based skills.

Most undergraduate medical programs have now identified the need to facilitate undergraduate education in inter-professional teams. The World Health Organization (WHO) defines inter-professional education as the process by which a group of students or workers from the health-related occupations with different backgrounds learn together during certain periods of their education, "with interaction as the important goal, to collaborate in providing promotive, preventive, curative, rehabilitative, and other health-related services"[17]. The medical manager is well placed to promote such team-based learning and team based care in the health services.

## Team Roles

Team based care requires medical managers to be aware of team composition and differing team roles. Meredith Belbin [18] described the behaviour of managers engaged in complex group exercises and found different personality traits styles and behaviours emerged. As time progressed different successful clusters of behaviour were identified. Belbin team roles describe the pattern of behaviour that characterises an individual's activities in relationship to another in facilitating the progress of the team's goals. The value of Belbin team-role theory lies in enabling individuals to evaluate and adjust individual behaviours according to the demands being made on the team. Belbin described three action oriented roles (shaper, implementer, completer), three people oriented roles (coordinator, team worker and resource Investigator) and three cerebral roles (innovator, monitor and evaluator). Whilst the team performs better if all nine Belbin roles are active, this is not always possible. The team leader's role is to recognise and correct for any of the groups deficits.

It is also important to realise that teams are dynamic units that are constantly changing. Tuckman [19] describes a series of stages through which a team travels as it forms and then achieves its goal (forming, storming, norming or performing). The medical manager needs to know which stage his or her team is at so that he/she can provide the necessary leadership. During the forming stage, individual roles and responsibilities are unclear and the medical manager must be prepared to clearly articulate these as well as address concerns about the team's purpose, objectives and external relationships. During the storming stage team members may become conflicted as they attempt to establish themselves in relation to others. During this phase the manager needs to be focused on the team goals to avoid becoming distracted. During the third, norming stage, agreement and consensus prevail as roles and responsibilities become clear and decisions begin to be made by the group through consensus. During this phase group unity and commitment is high and the leadership style can be less directed. In the final performing stage, the team has a shared vision and is able to operate with a high degree of autonomy.

## Consumer Consultation

Team based care should also involve regular consultation with all stakeholders including consumer consultation. The medical manager is encouraged to regularly look for opportunities to engage with consumer groups. It is critical to monitor and respond where appropriate to community perceptions about the quality of care the service provides. Community representation on hospital committees with responsibilities for governance and evaluation is recommended.

Patient centred care is health care that is respectful of, and responsive to, the preferences, needs and values of patients and consumers. There is growing evidence that partnerships between health service providers and patients, families, carers and consumers, benefits clinical quality and outcomes as well as the experience of care. Such benefits include decreased mortality [20] decreased readmission rates [21], decreased rates of healthcare acquired infections [22] reduced length of stay [23] and improved compliance regimens [24]. Additional benefits to the organisation include increased workforce satisfaction and retention rates [25]. The medical manager's role is to create a work environment that is responsive to patient, carer and consumer input and needs. Active partnership with consumers by health service organisations is key. Governance structures need to be in place which supports partnerships with consumers and/or carers. Such involvement can include decision making about safety and quality initiatives and quality improvement activities as well as consumers and/or carer feedback on patient information publications prepared by the health service for distribution to patients. This support typically extends to the organisation providing orientation and ongoing training for consumers and/or carers to enable them to fulfil their partnership role. Medical leaders should also ensure ongoing training is available to clinical and other managers on the value of and ways to facilitate consumer engagement and how to best create and sustain partnerships.

In summary, medical managers need to be able to effectively lead and participate in healthcare teams to achieve optimal patient care. This is increasingly important in a modern multi-professional environment, where the patient-centred care is shared across a variety of health care providers. Modern healthcare teams not only include group of professionals working closely together at one site, but also extend to teams operating in multiple locations. The potential for conflict is ever present and it is therefore essential for medical managers to be able to prevent, negotiate, and resolve inter-professional conflict.

# Case Study 1

You are the newly appointed Director of Paediatric Services in a largely rural area. You are aware that there has been a cluster of drug overdoses in young people from the local secondary schools and you decide to contact the local adolescent mental health services manager and community drop in centres. You are informed that there is a concerning growing culture of use of party drugs through a local ring leader using social media. The adolescent mental health services manager is surprised to hear from you as previous request for meetings with your predecessor were ignored. She had sent a letter 6 months ago requesting an interdisciplinary approach to the management of adolescent health to your predecessor but had not received a reply.

The local newspaper has recently run a front page story entitled "Drugs and Our Teenagers?" which includes an editorial highly critical of the local medical services in addressing the problem.

The Chief Medical Officer requests an urgent meeting to discuss short, medium and long term responses to this crisis.

**Who are the key stakeholders?**
**What are the main issues emerging?**
**What options would you explore?**
Consider the following:

- Managing a potential public health crisis
- Restoring the relationship with allied health care providers and setting up for future regular dialogue
- Recognising the need for team based approach and the coordination of multiple agency services
- Examination of any Coronial findings and recommendations from the earlier deaths
- Liaise with other primary care providers
- Liaise with schools
- Check with your own Emergency Department
- What services are available services for young adults, are there identifiable gaps in service provision

- Consider establishing a 'road show' in schools educating the students about the risks
- Consider community participation and consultation to address any local issues
- Consider responding to the critical editorial in the paper with the assistance of media advisors

## Case Study 2

You are the Medical Administrator in a hospital providing interventional radiology services. You were on the selection committee for the recently appointed interventional radiologist and are hoping his department can generate the savings alluded to at his interview. Your director of nursing rings you the minute you arrive to work to discuss special training needs for staff "if they are going to be called routinely to assist afterhours the new interventional radiologist". You recall a memo from the Head of Radiology requesting after hours support for proposed ablation therapies to commence next month. As you glance down at your diary you see you also have an appointment to meet with the Business Manager of the Radiology department and later in the day the Clinical Governance Unit Director.

The Business manager is concerned he is having 'some issues' with the newly appointed interventional radiologist, Dr X, who is insisting the purchase of three costly microwave ablation devices be approved. The radiologist was reportedly verbally aggressive to the Business Manager when his requests were denied, claiming that this is a new technique which has been available overseas for several months. The interventional radiologist claims he has received dedicated training in this new procedure, which is expected to generate significant savings for the hospital through reduced lengths of stay. He cannot understand why the hospital i.e. the business manager was putting obstacles in his way by insisting he make a formal written application before commencing the new procedure.

During your meeting with the Director of the Clinical Governance Unit, you find she has heard through the grapevine that the hospital is introducing new techniques in microwave ablation through the radiology department. She understands the rationale for the procedure however has concerns about undertaking new procedures without it having been through the hospital "Safety and Efficacy Register of New Interventional Procedures". She also tells you that the Hospital Foundation has already agreed to donate a significant sum of money to the Radiology department as a result of the Dr Xs "impressive" presentation to the Foundation and Consumer Reference Group meeting last month.

**What are the main issues?**

**Who are the key stakeholders?**

**What will you do in the short term and in the mid to long term?**

**What can you do to improve collaboration?**

- Involvement of key stakeholders
- Induction of new staff
- All new procedure needs special application to provide quality and timely assessments of new and emerging technologies and techniques (Consider evidence base, justification, outcomes, complications, patient selection, who will undertake, support requirements, follow up, evaluation, cost, benefit, timing, governance)
- Immediate advice – likely that Dr X defer procedure until formally approved
- New procedures require links with hospital strategic plans
- Deal with potential conflict between radiologist and business manager
- Quality and Safety – why so expensive?
- Opportunity for consumer reference group collaboration
- Opportunity to further engage Hospital foundation once new procedures approved
- Credentialling issues – how many procedures per year
- Accreditation processes? College guidelines

# References

1. Freeman T. Comparing the content of leadership theories and managers' shared perceptions of effective leadership: a Q method study of trainee managers in the English NHS. Health Serv Manage Res. 2013;26:43–53.

2. Fulop L, Mark A. Relational leadership, decision-making and the messiness of context in healthcare. Leadership. 2013;9(2):254–77.

3. Cunliffe AL, Eriksen M. Relational leadership. Hum Relations. 2011;64(11):1425–49.

4. Weick KE. Sensemaking in organizations, Foundations for organizational science. Thousand Oaks: Sage Publications; 1995. xii, 231.

5. Boje DM. Narrative methods for organizational and communication research, SAGE series in management research. London/ Thousand Oaks: Sage; 2001. p. 152.

6. MacCarrick G. Curriculum reform: a narrated journey. Med Educ. 2009;43(10):979–88.

7. Czarniawska B. Narrating the organization: dramas of institutional identity, New practices of inquiry. Chicago: University of Chicago Press; 1997. vii, 233.

8. Czarniawska B. Narrative interviews and organisations. In: Gubrium JH, Holstein JA, editors. Handbook of interview research: context and method. Thousand Oaks: Sage; 2002.

9. Thomas WI, Znaniecki F. The Polish peasant in Europe and America, vol. 2. New York: Knopf; 1927.

10. Polkinghorne D. Narrative knowing and the human sciences, SUNY series in philosophy of the social sciences. Albany: State University of New York Press; 1988. xi, 232.

11. Boje DM. The storytelling organization: a study of story performance in an office-supply firm. Adm Sci Q. 1991;36(1):106–26.

12. Ivancevich JM, Matteson MT, Olekalns M. Organisational behaviour and management. 1st Australasian ed. Sydney: Irwin; 1997. xx, 752.

13. Pondy LR. Organizational conflict: concepts and models. Adm Sci Q. 1967;12(2):296–320.

14. Hammick M, Olckers L, Campion-Smith C. Learning in interprofessional teams: AMEE Guide no 38. Med Teach. 2009;31(1):1–12.

15. McNair RP. The case for educating health care students in professionalism as the core content of interprofessional education. Med Educ. 2005;39(5):456–64.

16. Leavitt M. Medscape's response to the Institute of Medicine Report: crossing the quality chasm: a new health system for the 21st century. MedGenMed. 2001;3(2):2.
17. World Health Organisation. Learning together to work together for health. Report of a WHO Study Group on Multiprofessional Education of Health Personnel: the Team Approach. World Health Organ Tech Rep Ser. 1988;769:1–72.
18. Belbin RM. Team roles at work. Oxford: Boston: Butterworth-Heinemann; 1993. vii, 152.
19. Tuckman BW. Developmental sequence in small groups. Psychol Bull. 1965;63:84–9.
20. Meterko M, Wright S, Lin H, Lowy E, Cleary PD. Mortality among patients with acute myocardial infarction: the influences of patient-centered care and evidence-based medicine. Health Serv Res. 2010;45(5 Pt 1):1188–204.
21. Boulding W, Glickman SW, Manary MP, Schulman KA, Staelin R. Relationship between patient satisfaction with inpatient care and hospital readmission within 30 days. Am J Manag Care. 2011;17(1):41–8.
22. Edgcumbe DP. Patients' perceptions of hospital cleanliness are correlated with rates of meticillin-resistant Staphylococcus aureus bacteraemia. J Hosp Infect. 2009;71(1):99–101.
23. DiGioia A, Greenhouse PK, Levison TJ. Patient and family-centered collaborative care: an orthopaedic model. Clin Orthop Relat Res. 2007;463:13–9.
24. Arbuthnott A, Sharpe D. The effect of physician-patient collaboration on patient adherence in non-psychiatric medicine. Patient Educ Couns. 2009;77(1):60–7.
25. Charmel PA, Frampton SB. Building the business case for patient-centered care. Healthc Financ Manage. 2008;62(3):80–5.

# Chapter 7
# The Active Advocate

**Abstract** The medical manager as health advocate uses their expertise and influence to advance the health and well-being of individual patients, communities, and populations.

**Keywords** Determinants of health • Health promotion • Resource allocation

## Active Health Advocate

The medical practitioner is constantly confronted by the adverse effects of social inequality on the health of patients and communities. The challenge for the medical manager is to respond effectively to these [1]. The Canadian Medical Education Directions for Specialists (CanMEDS) framework includes health advocacy as a key component [2]. The role of a health advocate, as described in the CanMEDS 2005 framework, is defined as "physicians (who) responsibly use their expertise and influence to advance the health and well-being of individual patients, communities, and populations". Similarly, the American Medical Association declaration of professional responsibility states that physicians must "advocate for the social, economic, educational, and political changes that ameliorate suffering and contribute to human well-being" [3].

G. MacCarrick, *Medical Leadership and Management:*
*A Case-based Approach*, DOI 10.1007/978-1-4471-4748-0_7,
© Springer-Verlag London 2014

The relevant competencies, required of the active health advocate include:

- Ability to respond to individual patient health needs and issues
- Ability to respond to the health needs of the communities they serve particularly marginalised populations
- Describe and identify the determinants of health of the populations they serve
- Commitment to promoting the health of individual patients, communities and populations
- Understands the ethics of resource allocation
- Ability to influence policy and practice to improve health outcomes

It has been argued that the medical profession has not always accepted calls for greater public engagement owing to the increasing demands and practice changes. While most physicians recognize the importance of working on public health and population health issues, many are not [1, 4–6]. Gruen and colleagues argue that if calls for public engagement by doctors are to be effective then there must be "a clear and justifiable definition" of the roles of the health advocate with articulation of reasonable limits as to what can be expected which are compatible with busy practice [6] (p 94).

The model Gruen and colleagues describe includes three domains of professional obligation and two domains of professional aspiration. Doctors have professional obligations to promotion access to care and address socio-economic factors that influence directly an individuals' health (for example smoking). Aspirations for improved health outcomes (education, opportunity health inequities) whilst laudable may not be sufficiently different from the aspirations of other citizens in the community and as such are considered domains of professional aspiration. At the centre of the model is the doctor's responsibility to provide high quality care to individual patients. Outside the core responsibility of individual patient care is the impact that access to care has on health. Factors that influence access include for example, availability of after-hours care, geographic distribution of services, access for disabled and indigenous patients. The framework described by Gruen and colleagues is useful in defining where the boundary should exist between professional obligation and professional aspiration. The medical manager has a particular role in promoting systems of care that ensure all patients have access to appropriate health care. Medical managers have a responsibility to work with other colleagues in addressing the causes of poor access and also have a responsibility to become involved in addressing socio-economic factors that are associated directly with poor health outcomes.

Six attributes of the health advocate have been described namely being knowledgeable, altruistic, honest, assertive, resourceful, and up-to date [7]. As knowledgeable health advocates, managers need to be familiar with the major issues in current public policy and be able to articulate priorities and opportunities to improve quality of care. Medical managers also need to be able to obtain and demonstrate the application of unbiased information. Managers must also understand the ethics of resource allocation as well as barriers to access to care and resources.

There is ample literature verifying ethnic differences in physical health, with most pointing to poorer health outcomes in ethnic minorities. The influence of social factors such as low socio-economic status and deprivation has also been shown, [8, 9]. The medical manager needs to be familiar with all aspects of population health including reliable tools for measurement of the burden of disease as well as measurement of risk and vulnerability. In mental health for example one such tool is the Health of the Nation Outcome Scales (HoNOS) [10], providing professionals with a systematic summary which is easy to use and provides consistent measurements and outcome information which allows staff to work with the same set of criteria.

By using integrated clinical information systems, the health care manager can advocate for improved coordination of services by different agencies. Simple strategies such as improved agreement on definitions of common clinical terms, actions and outcomes within disciplines and across different agencies can lead to improved health outcomes. The health care manager has a particular role to play in promoting standardisation in the way clinical information is defined, gathered and coded.

In summary as active advocates, medical managers use their clinical and management expertise to influence policy and practice to advance the health and well-being of individual patients, communities, and populations.

# Case Study 1

You are the Director of Medical Services of a public hospital which serves a mixed rural and urban population of 350,000 people. You and your team are reviewing your strategic plan for your services with the aim of better meeting the needs of your catchment population in the short and longer term within your existing budget.

Recently your CEO has been challenged in the press and at a public forum by a local Indigenous elder, who claims that Indigenous people do not have the same access to health care services at your hospital as non- indigenous persons, drawing attention to the Prime Minister's announced commitment to Indigenous people under the "Close the Gap" strategy.

You know that some Indigenous people are ageing earlier than the general population, in terms of diabetes and obesity-related hypertension. There is also over-representation in the prevalence of mental health disorders amongst your Indigenous peoples.

Your CEO wants some briefing notes from you for urgent circulation to Board members before their next monthly meeting.

Your recall a recent presentation in which Health of the Nation Outcome Scale (HoNOS) data was presented at a subcommittee meeting on mental health care in your region.

**What are the key points that will be included in your briefing?**

- Identify the current situation
- What proportion of population is indigenous?
- Baseline patterns of morbidity and mortality
- Prevalence of diabetes, hypertension and obesity in local indigenous group
- Prevalence of complications in different sub-populations
- Identify existing services? In hospital, in community health, in GP surgeries, in non-gov organisations for indigenous people
- What are the gaps in services?
- Identified special advisory group including representation from local indigenous group
- Refer to relevant Indigenous Health Strategy
- Any plan should be consistent with national strategies and must satisfy the needs as perceived by the local indigenous groups as well as ensure that resources are equitably distributed.
- What model of care is best? – May be cultural requirement to care for families/elders at home as much as possible
- Best model likely to be a community based program, with large component of targeted health promotion activities.

# Case Study 2

You are the newly appointed CEO of a district health service for a region covering 250,000 population. The district health service includes three hospitals, two nursing homes and several community health units. Your focus during the previous 6 months has been attempting to manage the service within a policy of tight fiscal constraint. Although you have had some success overall this has been a very challenging period. Now as you start a new year a change of government has been announced and with it a renewed focus on population health. The hospital board want you to move the service from its current focus of acute hospital care towards a more integrated population health approach. You have been invited to draft a strategic planning framework to achieve this goal.

**What are the features of the two different approaches? What are the challenges you expect to face?**

- A service managed under primarily economic parameters has a focus on: cost cutting measures, throughput indicators, rationing, priority setting and capping demand.
- A service managed under a primarily population health approach has a focus on: population health indicators, health promotion and early intervention, health versus treatment services and different timelines.
- Anticipate challenges with different stakeholder groups, such as funder, purchaser and provider divisions.
- What theoretical framework to use to effect change management and managing resistance to change
- Establishing a realistic timeframe with specific achievable goals and measurable outcomes
- Improved integration between primary health care and acute treatment services
- Responding to the health needs of the community especially marginalised populations
- Ethics of resource allocation
- Creating a learning organization

## References

1. Furler J, et al. Health inequalities, physician citizens and professional medical associations: an Australian case study. BMC Med. 2007;5:23.
2. Frank JR, Danoff D. The CanMEDS initiative: implementing an outcomes-based framework of physician competencies. Med Teach. 2007;29(7):642–7.

3. American Medical Association. Declaration of professional responsibility: medicine's social contract with humanity. Available from: http://www.med.illinois.edu/depts_programs/ ClinicalAffairs/Document/decofprofessional.pdf. Cited 10 Apr 2014.

4. Gruen RL, Campbell EG, Blumenthal D. Public roles of US physicians: community participation, political involvement, and collective advocacy. JAMA. 2006;296(20):2467–75.

5. Brill JR, Ohly S, Stearns MA. Training community-responsive physicians. Acad Med. 2002;77(7):747.

6. Gruen RL, Pearson SD, Brennan TA. Physician-citizens–public roles and professional obligations. JAMA. 2004;291(1):94–8.

7. Flynn L, Verma S. Fundamental components of a curriculum for residents in health advocacy. Med Teach. 2008;30(7):e178–83.

8. Schoenbaum M, Waidmann T. Race, socioeconomic status, and health: accounting for race differences in health. J Gerontol B Psychol Sci Soc Sci. 1997;52 Spec No:61–73.

9. Franks P, Gold MR, Fiscella K. Sociodemographics, self-rated health, and mortality in the US. Soc Sci Med. 2003;56(12):2505–14.

10. Wing JK, et al. Health of the Nation Outcome Scales (HoNOS). Research and development. Br J Psychiatry. 1998;172:11–8.

# Chapter 8
# The Resourceful Scholar

**Abstract** Managers must demonstrate lifelong commitment to self-directed learning which includes critically evaluating information for decision making; facilitating learning for all stakeholders and applying research skills to management tasks.

**Keywords** Self- directed learning • Critical appraisal • Educational theory • Ethical research • Research governance

## Resourceful Scholar

Modern medical practitioners are expected to demonstrate lifelong commitment to learning as well as to the development and communication of new knowledge. Most medical competency frameworks in current use across the globe contain statements of outcome relating to scholarship and evidence-based practice. In their Scholar role [1], doctors are expected to demonstrate a lifelong commitment to reflective learning, as well as the creation, dissemination, application and translation of medical knowledge [2]. Specific scholar competencies in relation to the medical managers' role are that the medical manager critically evaluate information for decision making; facilitate learning for all stakeholders and demonstrate the ability to apply research skills to management tasks.

G. MacCarrick, *Medical Leadership and Management:*
*A Case-based Approach*, DOI 10.1007/978-1-4471-4748-0_8,
© Springer-Verlag London 2014

The relevant competencies required of the resourceful scholar include:

- Consistently demonstrates maintenance of ongoing self- directed learning
- Ability to research, collate and critically appraise information for decision making
- Supports and facilitates teaching and learning including of peers, trainees, colleagues and other stakeholders
- Understands underlying principles of educational theory and research
- Adheres to principles of ethical research
- Provides leadership of effective research governance

## Medical Managers as Teachers

Medical managers are very well placed to ensure a work climate in which education, training and research can flourish [3, 4] and are well placed to take some responsibility for teaching management competencies. Supporting professional development in a distributed leadership model builds what Day calls the 'social capital' of the organization [5]. Recent studies have shown that doctors in training do not feel fully prepared in terms of perceived management competencies despite the incorporation of the CanMEDS framework into most medical curricula [6, 7]. Yet most junior doctors feel that receiving formal management training positively influences perceived management competencies. These studies clearly indicate a role for medical managers as teachers to help embed relevant management and leadership competencies in both the undergraduate and postgraduate setting medical education setting. Many teachers and trainers involved in educating in the clinical setting are not only involved with undergraduate medical education i.e. medical students, but are also trainers and supervisors of postgraduate trainees.

In most jurisdictions, medical school graduate outcome statements emphasise the importance of the doctor's role as teacher. The Australian Medical Council statement emphasizes the wider scholarly role doctors can play in teaching, assessing and providing feedback and evaluation:

> On entry to professional practice, Australian and New Zealand graduates are able to...... communicate effectively in wider roles including health advocacy, teaching, assessing and appraising [8] (page 3).

The CanMEDS Competency Framework is not only a useful way to consider the knowledge, skills and abilities that doctors need to deliver better patient outcomes, but it can also be used as a way of conceptualizing good clinical teaching [9]. Prideaux and colleagues [9] maintain that clinical teaching is at the centre of medical education. Traditionally clinical teaching has taken place in large teaching hospitals or academic medical centres [10]. Increasingly the pattern of teaching is changing as the patient mix in teaching hospitals changes as well as demography, ageing populations, patient expectations, developments in disease treatments and information technology. As more care is being delivered in the ambulatory or community based setting, medical managers need to be aware of the implications for teaching resource management and distribution. In the midst of this change there is ongoing concern about competing demands between teaching and service provision, which presents another particular challenge for the medical manager.

Medical managers will typically be involved in support of a variety of educational programs for junior and senior doctors. Engagement with local Medical Education Units, support of post-graduate medical education and supervision for junior doctors; support of specialist training posts as well as generic education and training such as computer and management skills; clinical skills sessions (including Grand rounds, morbidity/mortality review sessions); skills development centres as well as general oversight of professional development leave for doctors are all part of the medical manager's brief. The medical manager's role often extends to oversight of quarantined time for dedicated teaching. In this capacity the manager can influence recognition of the value of teaching and raise its priority. Some medical professional organisations have gone so far as to issue guidance on recognition of teaching responsibilities in service job descriptions [11].

Apart from the support of teaching, medical managers should be skilled as teachers themselves. By modelling personal educational strategies such as self-directed learning, managers provide powerful examples for their trainees to follow. They can also assist trainees in facilitating self-direction in learning through assistance with goal setting and feedback. Managers as scholars locate, appraise and apply best available evidence to inform their own management practice. Making this explicit is a powerful teaching tool [12, 13]. Managers should also teach in a manner which recognizes the different educational needs of different learner groups, as well as the different learning style [14, 15]. Both Ullian et al. and Irby claim that effective teachers are those that act as role models and are also supportive supervisors. It stands to reason that the same can be said of medical managers who teach and supervise trainees in the discipline of medical management and leadership.

Peer Review of Learning and Teaching (PRLT) is another area in which medical managers can become involved. This typically formative process encourages clinician teachers to reflect on their teaching and ensures that they receive feedback from colleagues. There exists a need to ensure the recognition of all teaching and training in job plans and to quality assures this in the same way as any other consultant activity. While processes will vary between employers, appraisals of those with roles in teaching should include the educational activities they undertake, as suggested in *Tomorrow's Doctors* (2009):

> Appraisals should cover teaching responsibilities for all relevant consultant, academic and other staff, whether or not employed by the university.

The result of the teaching performance evaluation and 360° feedback, together with the teacher's personal reflection, should feed into appraisal. The outcome can inform the educational elements of the teacher's personal development plan and will enable the performance manager to target training and resources where it is needed.

One of the most notable findings in the early work of Irby and colleagues (above) showed clustering of items associated with learner autonomy i.e. respecting the autonomy of the learner and nurturing self-directed learning appear to be key elements of teaching effectiveness [13]. An effective strategy for the manager as teacher, particularly in the post graduate setting is relational teaching [16]. In relational teaching the perspective on teaching and learning becomes a two-way inter-action, in which students and the teacher become co-learners. A relational view of learning sees the how and the what of learning as inseparable aspects of learning [17]. It conceptu-alises the teaching and learning process holistically. Describes relational pedagogy in which students are encouraged to develop more sophisticated ways of knowing by providing learning experiences that relate to prior experiences, facilitat-ing a constructivist perspective on knowing and learning, and providing opportunities for learners to access peer perspec-tives [18]. Relational teaching involves inquiry into how stu-dents learn, encouraging teachers, like trainees to be critically reflective life-long learners. Ongoing faculty development, delivered by educationalists therefore has a significant role to play in providing methodological advice and support to teach-ers engaged in relational teaching. Typically the coordination of the delivery of appropriate staff development is the realm of Departments of Medical Education [19, 20] and in some jurisdictions such departments are affiliated with tertiary care settings. The Medical Education Unit typically falls under the remit of the Director of Medical Services.

# Medical Managers as Curriculum Planners

Outcomes-based education has influenced many modern day medical curricula as a means of making explicit to trainees what specific knowledge, attitudes and skills they will acquire by the end of training and by the end of each unit of study [9]. Using an 'outcomes focused' approach in embedding competencies in medical leadership and management ensures the learning journey is signposted for trainees and faculty. Students can more readily make links between the desired knowledge skills and attitudes and the teaching, learning and assessment strategies used. Biggs coined the term "constructive alignment" [9–12]:

> In aligned teaching, there is maximum consistency throughout the system. The curriculum is stated in the form of clear objectives, which state the level of understanding required rather than simply a list of topics to be covered. The teaching methods are chosen that are likely to realise these objectives...the assessment tasks address the objectives... students are "entrapped" in this web of consistency. (Biggs p. 27)

In defining curriculum outcomes a medical management and leadership curriculum should be derived in consultation with relevant stakeholders who are cognizant of the various health care settings in which the candidates will work. The Medical Leadership Competency Framework (MLCF) [21] for example was jointly developed by the Academy of Medical Royal Colleges and the NHS Institute for Innovation and Improvement, in conjunction with a wide range of stakeholders. Also consulted were members of the medical and wider NHS community including reference and focus groups. Likewise the RACMA curriculum project was informed by an 18-month cross-disciplinary, collaborative and consultative process involving Fellows, Associate Fellows, and Candidates, other specialist colleagues, academics and community members. Regular review of curriculum outcomes by specialist Colleges such as these ensures the necessary linkage between outcomes and assessment and that the curriculum reflects latest and best practice in medical management and leadership.

## Medical Managers as Assessors

There are several key principles to consider if the medical manager becomes involved in assessment of students or trainees. The focus of assessment should be on judging student mastery of knowledge, skills and attitudes, measuring improvement over time, diagnosing student difficulties and motivating students. The strategy should also focus on learning to take responsibility for owns one ongoing life- long learning and professional development. A focus for assessors and teachers should be to provide high quality formative (see below) assessment, through regular feedback. The purpose of each component of the assessment should be clearly defined for students and trainees, ensuring the content derives from and represents the breadth of the curriculum. The assessment strategies chosen must be valid and reliable. Importantly the assessment should reflect the educational objectives of the curriculum and be capable of identifying trainees/students who are under-performing and possibly in need of remediation. Most Colleges will have an assessment policy document which informs faculty and students about all matters relating to assessment. This will typically contain information such as the assessment blueprint [22] which will ensure that each assessment is based on appropriate sampling of the program learning outcomes. The assessment policy should also describe the basis for and timing of formative[1] and summative[2] assessments; rules related to attendance; the different types of knowledge based and performance based assessments in use; process for managing poorly performing and fitness to practice issues such as health or personal issues and professionalism. Medical student and trainee assessment of management and leadership competencies should include direct observation of skills, behaviours, and attitudes that have been specified in the educational objectives of the program.

There should also be regular assessment of problem solving, decision making, and communication skills. It should be clear to all stakeholders how each component of the curriculum is being assessed. Table 8.1 shows how the RACMA Scholar competence is assessed using a variety of different strategies

---

[1] Formative assessment is intended to modify and to inform student learning. Formative methods of assessment generally precede a summative assessment method and are not part of the official student record of achievement.

[2] Summative assessment evaluates mastery of the learning objectives of the course, forms part or all of the final result and determines progression within the course.

TABLE 8.1 Excerpt from The RACMA medical leadership and management curriculum: role competency – scholar (Reproduced with permission)

| Role competencies | Key goals | Workplace activities | Novice | Apprentice | Competent | Assessment |
|---|---|---|---|---|---|---|
| Scholar | Maintain and enhance professional activities through ongoing learning | Actively participate in an organisational quality committee, preferably the peak executive or Board quality committee. | Participate in an organisational quality committee. | Actively participate in an organisational quality committee. | Actively participate in an organisational quality committee, preferably the peak executive or Board quality committee. | Health Service Evaluation research project |
| | | Participate in individual and organisation-sponsored continuing professional education. Attend skill development workshops, courses and keep up to date with relevant literature. | Participate in individual and organisation-sponsored continuing professional education. | Participate in individual and organisation-sponsored continuing professional education. | Participate in individual and organisation-sponsored continuing professional education. Attend skill development workshops, courses and keep up to date with relevant literature. | Oral presentation of research project |

| | | | | |
|---|---|---|---|---|
| Be involved in one or more of: | Attend skill development workshops, courses and keep up to date with relevant literature. | Attend skill development workshops, courses and keep up to date with relevant literature. | Be involved in one or more of: | In-training assessment reports |
| Clinical Risk Management training or activities | Undertake a quality improvement activity. | Be involved in one or more of: | Clinical Risk Management training or activities | Leadership case study |
| Review of a clinical incident | | Clinical Risk Management training or activities | Review of a clinical incident. | |
| Undertake or lead a quality improvement activity. | | Review of a clinical incident. | Lead a quality improvement activity. | |
| Keep up to date with clinical developments relevant to the organization. | | Undertake or lead a quality improvement activity. | | |

including submission of a research project, an oral presentation of research conducted as well as a leadership case study.

As teachers responsible for curriculum delivery, medical managers should understand the purposes and benefits of different types of assessment and the uses and limitations of various test formats. For instance criterion-referenced vs. norm-referenced assessment and formative vs. summative assessment. For example assessing knowledge may be achieved using multiple choice questions [23], extended matching items [24], key features testing [25] or constructed response questions [26]. Assessing skills may be achieved using OSCEs [27] and measurement of acquisition of appropriate attributes such as professionalism can be explored using portfolios [28]. Van der Vleuten [29] describes five helpful criteria for determining the usefulness of a particular method of assessment: reliability (the degree to which the measurement is accurate and reproducible), validity (whether the assessment measures what it claims to measure), impact on future learning and practice, acceptability to learners and faculty, and the cost of assessment. This is a useful framework for medical managers to conceptualise any assessment strategy which is being used to measure mastery of management and leadership competence.

## Medical Managers as Researchers

Developing a scientific mind is an important part of the role of manager. The ability to appraise and apply scientific evidence is key. Trainees of most medical Colleges are expected to demonstrate a lifelong commitment to learning as well as to the development and communication of new knowledge. For the medical manager this applies to not only best clinical practice but also to medical leadership and management practice. The most relevant form of research involving medical managers is that which explores health services.

Health Services Research is typically a multi-disciplinary research activity which has an emphasis on improving health services. The Health Services Research Association of Australia and New Zealand (HSRAANZ) [30] make the important distinction between Health Services Research (HSR) and single-discipline research in that HSR seeks to understand dimensions of health services from multiple perspectives. As such, medical managers can draw on theoretical frameworks from a variety of disciplines including medicine, nursing, allied health, psychology, sociology, political science, management science and health economics.

HSRAANZ also make the point that HSR is an area of "applied rather than 'basic'" research, using theories of human behaviour from contributing disciplines to generate and test hypotheses about the delivery of health care. Improvement of health services has many dimensions, including quality of care (effective, timely and appropriate); accessible care; equal distribution of health gains; safer care and more efficient care. Research however is often constrained by lack of resources and in particular, time. Even for trainers and curriculum planners integrating learning about research skills and methods into the curriculum is challenging [31] and many graduates are left lacking confidence in their ability to assess the worth of a research article or indeed how to go about generating a worthy research question to pursue.

A key to practicing evidence-based leadership in healthcare is being information literate. Recognising the need for information and determining the nature and extent of information needed; finding needed information effectively and efficiently; critically evaluating information and the information seeking process; managing information collected or generated; applying prior and new information to construct new concepts or create new understandings and acknowledging cultural, ethical, economic, legal and social issues surrounding the use of information are the key elements underpinning most information literacy standards.

In addition understanding the principals of ethical research is an important consideration for medical managers who will often be invited to join or lead ethics committees. Research is evaluated on several core principles. For instance, research is considered to have *merit* if it can be demonstrated to yield potential benefit, which may include its contribution to knowledge and understanding and improved social welfare and wellbeing. It must also be based upon methods appropriate for achieving the aims of the proposal and based on a thorough study of the current literature. The merit of a research proposal should also be based upon ensuring respect for the participants is not compromised; conducted or supervised by persons or teams with experience, qualifications and competence and conducted using facilities and resources appropriate for the research. Research is considered to have been conducted with *integrity* if it is carried out by researchers with a commitment to searching for and who are committed to disseminating this new knowledge and understanding and permit open and public scrutiny of all research findings. Research is considered to be *just*, if it is conducted in a fair manner for example if the selection process is fair and transparent, there is fair distribution of the benefits of participation in research and the outcomes are accessible to all research participants in a timely manner. Research is considered to be *beneficent* if the likely benefits of the project justify any risks of harm or discomfort to participants. Finally, research must preserve respect for human beings with due regard for the welfare, beliefs, perceptions, customs and cultural heritage, of those research participants. This includes maintenance of participant autonomy throughout the research process, including making the decision to withdraw at any time without any effect, should they wish.

These key principles are informed by legislation and guidelines, which the medical manager should be familiar with. These include statements and codes on ethical and responsible conduct in human research. Typically human research ethics committees are established by universities and hospitals to provide ethical oversight of human research including review of research proposals; monitoring the conduct of research; ensuring compliance with relevant standards and guidelines and dealing with complaints that arise from the conduct of research.

Medical Managers have a responsibility to ensure that any research involving their facilities, staff or patients, is transparent and accountable and meets the relevant legal, ethical and administrative requirements. Managers needs to be aware of the relevant legislation relating to matters such as the

Coroner's office, gene technology; guardianship and administration; mental health; public health and information privacy.

In summary, medical managers must demonstrate a life-long commitment to reflective learning, as well as the creation, dissemination, application and translation of new medical management knowledge. The particular discipline of health services research draws from a wide range of disciplines including the contributing direct service disciplines of medicine, nursing and allied health but also psychology, sociology, political science, management science and health economics. The overall improvement of health services includes dimensions such as quality of care (effective, timely and appropriate); accessibility of care; distribution of health gains; safe care and efficient care. The medical manager's role a scholar is to seek and disseminate greater understanding of these dimensions of health care from multiple perspectives.

# Case Study 1

You are the Director of Medical Services and a recently appointed member of the Human Research Ethics Committee of a large teaching hospital. Your trainee advises you that she has heard that the department of Medicine has commenced a large drug company funded trial of new anticoagulant therapy and is concerned as she had also heard that collection of baseline patient blood samples was occurring without patient consent.

**What are the ethical and clinical governance issues arising from this case?**

**How will you manage these?**

- Consider governance of research ethics and what mechanisms are or should be in place to oversee research in your hospital? Research Governance Officer, Human Research Ethics Committee
- Collect the facts.
- Has an approval been granted for this study?
- What consent issues were raised as part of the proposal?
- How was respect for participants to be ensured?

- Has there been a breach of the conduct?
- Discuss the underlying principles of ethical and responsible conduct of research in involving humans.

## Case Study 2

You are the Director of Medical Services at a large regional hospital. The Director of Emergency Department has come to see you to complain about the 'time-consuming' new resident evaluation forms he has been asked to complete by the Director of Clinical Training (DCT) and how he doesn't have the time to waste completing these, especially the 360° resident evaluations.

He also wishes to discuss the 'onerous teaching commitment' he has inherited from his predecessor (a much valued teacher and mentor at the hospital, now retired) as service delivery is his paramount concern with a recent blow out in Emergency Department waiting times.

**Discuss the key issues arising from this case?**
**How will you manage these?**

- Research the case in advance
- Meet with your DCT, what do the forms look like? how long to they actually take to complete?
- What is contained in the employment contracts for senior medical staff, does the contract stipulate dedicated teaching and if so how much time?
- Listen carefully to the ED Director's concerns.
- Do you feel the Director or her/his staff would benefit for up-skilling in teaching.
- Are there more effective ways of delivering the teaching?
- Remain committed to support for teaching and learning at your Hospital.
- Recognise the importance of both teaching and effective feedback to junior medical staff as a recruitment and retention tool especially in a regional setting which relies on returned workforce.

# Case Study 3

One of your Medical Management trainees is required to conduct a research project (not an audit) as part of her training and seeks your advice. She has considered using some existing retrospective data she found "sitting around" which looks at Hospital in the Home re-admission rates. She says she is struggling to make the distinction between audit and research. She also expresses concern that the Training program is trying to turn her into a researcher, when what she really wanted was to join a specialty that would specifically develop her management skills and focus more on the 'front-line, hands on management'.

**Discuss the key issues arising?**
**How will you best support your trainee?**

- Help make the distinction between audit and research – The intended outcome of audit is to document quality or where necessary to take steps to provide a better service, whereas the ultimate outcome of research is to improve knowledge.
- Results of audit tend to be only valid in the particular context, ie this hospital
- Discuss with candidate the characteristics of a good research question, using framework such as [32]: feasible, interesting, novel, ethical, and relevant
- Is the potential project feasible, are there adequate number of subjects, adequate technical expertise, affordable in time and money, manageable in scope
- Interesting and Novel, will it confirm, refute or extend previous findings
- Ethical, ie amenable to a study that a HREC will approve
- Relevant, to the scientific community, to clinical and health policy
- Discuss with the trainee the importance of the medical manager's role in pursuits of scholarly role including research and teaching as well as evidence based decision making

## Case Study 4

The Director of Grand Rounds has belatedly invited you as the newly appointed Director of Medical Services to address next week's monthly meeting. She apologises for the late notice, but hopes that you can accept the invitation as the director of paediatrics has a clashing commitment on that particular day. She also acknowledges that medical administration is rarely present at grand rounds but hopes this will not stand in the way of your accepting this invitation.

By the time the invitation arrives by email you notice you have been scheduled to speak at the end of the session (just before the free lunch provided) as the last in a series of three speakers for the lunchtime meeting. You also read that the invitation to this meeting includes not only doctors in training and their consultants, but medical students are also invited and expected to attend.

**Discuss the key issues and opportunities arising from this case?**

**How will you approach the task at hand?**

- Accept the invitation and use it as an opportunity to profile the discipline of Medical Management
- If possible, negotiate an earlier place in the proposed schedule (given the late notice)
- Identify previous topics covered in grand rounds and the proposed topics of other co-speakers
- Avoid duplicating content
- Identify the relevant learning needs of the potential audience and try to make links between other presentations
- Choose a relevant and interesting topic which will help profile your specialist area in context and in a favourable light (given it is your first presentation to this audience and important stakeholder group)
- Use the opportunity to encourage consideration of future career paths for junior doctors
- Consider and recognise prior learning of audience and plan learning objectives, (a discussion with the Director of Clinical Training may be helpful in planning your presentation)

- Define learning objectives using for example Bloom's taxonomy [33]
- Consider timing (start and finish times and time for questions), resources (for example availability of on site e.g. video players, OHPs, slide projector or whiteboard), identify any technical issues such as compatibility issues related to use of computers which will need to be dealt with in advance.
- Plan an evaluation. This might include a formal written evaluation form administered after the presentation asking the audience to comment on how well the learning objectives were met.
- Consider regular involvement with Grand Rounds as a means of engaging with the hospital's medical workforce.

# References

1. Frank J, Danoff D. The CanMEDS initiative: implementing an outcomes-based framework of physician competencies. Med Teach. 2007;29(7):642–7.
2. The Royal College of Physicians and Surgeons of Canada. CanMEDS physician competency framework. 2005. Available from: http://www.royalcollege.ca/public/canmeds/framework. Cited 20 Feb 2012.
3. Steinert Y, et al. A systematic review of faculty development initiatives designed to improve teaching effectiveness in medical education: BEME Guide No. 8. Med Teach. 2006;28(6):497–526.
4. McLean M, Cilliers F, Van Wyk JM. Faculty development: yesterday, today and tomorrow. Med Teach. 2008;30(6):555–84.
5. Day DV. Leadership development: a review in context. Leadersh Q. 2000;11(4):581.
6. Berkenbosch L, et al. Medical residents' perceptions of their competencies and training needs in health care management: an international comparison. BMC Med Educ. 2013;13:25.
7. Schoenmaker SG, et al. Victorian junior doctors' perception of their competency and training needs in healthcare management. Aust Health Rev. 2013;37(4):412–7.
8. Australian Medical Council Incorporated. Assessment and accreditation of medical schools: standards and procedures. Canberra: Australian Medical Council Incorporated; 2002.

9. Prideaux D, et al. Clinical teaching: maintaining an educational role for doctors in the new health care environment. Med Educ. 2000;34(10):820–6.
10. Skeff KM, Bowen JL, Irby DM. Protecting time for teaching in the ambulatory care setting. Acad Med. 1997;72(8):694–7.
11. Academy of Medical Sciences 2010. Redressing the balance: the status and valuation of teaching in academic careers in the biomedical sciences. In: Available: http://www.acmedsci.ac.uk/policy/policy-projects/redressing-the-balance-the-status-and-valuation-of-teaching-in-academic-careers/.
12. Ullian JA, Bland CJ, Simpson DE. An alternative approach to defining the role of the clinical teacher. Acad Med. 1994; 69(10):832–8.
13. Irby DM, et al. Characteristics of effective clinical teachers of ambulatory care medicine. Acad Med. 1991;66(1):54–5.
14. Chapman DM, Calhoun JG. Validation of learning style measures: implications for medical education practice. Med Educ. 2006;40(6):576–83.
15. Smits PBA, et al. Factors predictive of successful learning in postgraduate medical education. Med Educ. 2004;38(7):758–66.
16. Brownlee J. Teacher education students' epistemological beliefs: developing a relational model of teaching. Res Educ. 2004;72:1–17, R5.
17. Ramsden P. Improving teaching and learning in higher education: the case for a relational perspective. Stud Higher Educ. 1987;12(3):275–86.
18. Magolda MB. Epistemological development in graduate and professional education. Review of Higher Educ. 1996;19(3): 283–304.
19. Albanese MA, Dottl S, Nowacek GA. Offices of research in medical education: accomplishments and added value contributions. Teach Learn Med. 2001;13(4):258–67.
20. Davis MH, Karunathilake I, Harden RM. AMEE Education Guide no. 28: the development and role of departments of medical education. Med Teach. 2005;27(8):665–75.
21. The Academy of Medical Royal Colleges and the NHS Institute for Innovation and Improvement. Medical leadership competency framework. 2011. Available from: http://www.leadershipacademy.nhs.uk/wp-content/uploads/2012/11/NHSLeadership-Leadership-Framework-Medical-Leadership-Competency-Framework-3rd-ed.pdf.

22. Coderre S, Woloschuk W, McLaughlin K. Twelve tips for blue-printing. Med Teach. 2009;31(4):322–4.
23. Norcini JJ, et al. A comparison of knowledge, synthesis, and clinical judgment. Multiple-choice questions in the assessment of physician competence. Eval Health Prof. 1984;7(4):485–99.
24. Swanson DB, et al. Psychometric characteristics and response times for content-parallel extended-matching and one-best-answer items in relation to number of options. Acad Med. 2006;81(10 Suppl):S52–5.
25. Page G, Bordage G, Allen T. Developing key-feature problems and examinations to assess clinical decision-making skills. Acad Med. 1995;70(3):194–201.
26. Feletti GI, Engel CE. The modified essay question for testing problem-solving skills. Med J Aust. 1980;1(2):79–80.
27. Harden RM. Twelve tips for organizing an Objective Structured Clinical Examination (OSCE). Med Teach. 1990;12(3–4):259–64.
28. Friedman Ben David M, et al. AMEE medical education guide no. 24: portfolios as a method of student assessment. Med Teach. 2001;23(6):535–51.
29. Van der Vleuten CP. The assessment of professional competence: developments, research and practical implications. Adv Health Sci Educ Theory Pract. 1996;1(1):41–67.
30. Health Services Research Association of Australia and New Zealand. What is HSR 2009. Available from: http://www.hsraanz.org/Home.aspx. Cited Feb 2014.
31. Mac Carrick G, Owen K, Hearder R. Preparing evidence based future medical leaders: an Australasian perspective. Asia Pac J Health Manag. 2014;9(1):14–7.
32. Hulley SB, Browner WS, Cummings SR. Designing clinical research: an epidemiologic approach. Baltimore/London: Williams & Wilkins; 1988. xi, 247 p.
33. Bloom B, Englehart M, Furst E, Hill W, Krathwohl D. Taxonomy of educational objectives: The classification of educational goals. Handbook I: Cognitive domain, New York, Toronto Longmans, Green. 1956.

# Index

G. MacCarrick, *Medical Leadership and Management:*          107
*A Case-based Approach*, DOI 10.1007/978-1-4471-4748-0,
© Springer-Verlag London 2014